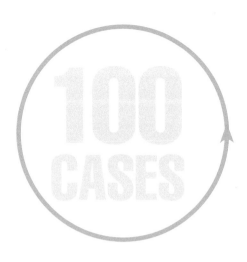

in
Obstetrics
and
Gynaecology

100 Cases in Obstetrics and Gynaecology presents 100 obstetric- or gynaecology-related scenarios commonly seen by medical students and junior doctors in the emergency department, outpatient clinic or on the ward. A succinct summary of the patient's history, examination and initial investigations – including photographs where relevant – is followed by questions on the diagnosis and management of each case. The answer includes a detailed discussion on each topic, with further illustration where appropriate, providing an essential revision aid as well as a practical guide for students and junior doctors.

Making speedy and appropriate clinical decisions, and choosing the best course of action to take as a result, is one of the most important and challenging parts of training to become a doctor. These true-to-life cases, fully revised and updated for this third edition, will teach students and junior doctors to recognize important obstetric and gynaecological conditions, and to develop their diagnostic and management skills.

100 Cases
About the Series

Making speedy and appropriate clinical decisions and choosing the best course of action to take as a result is one of the most important and challenging parts of training to become a doctor. The real-life cases presented in the 100 Cases series encompass emergency, ward, and outpatient and community scenarios, and have been designed specifically to help medical students and junior doctors to develop their diagnostic and management skills.

100 Cases in Dermatology
Rachael Morris-Jones, Ann-Marie Powell, Emma Benton

100 Cases in Radiology
Robert Thomas, James Connelly, Christopher Burke

100 Cases in Orthopaedics and Rheumatology
Parminder J Singh, Catherine Swales

100 Cases in Surgery, 2E
James Gossage, Bijan Modarai, Arun Sahai, Richard Worth, Kevin G Burnand

100 Cases in Clinical Ethics and Law, 2E
Carolyn Johnston, Penelope Bradbury

100 Cases in Paediatrics, 2E
Ronny Cheung, Aubrey Cunnington, Simon Drysdale, Joseph Raine, Joanna Walker

100 Cases in General Practice, 2E
Anne E Stephenson, Martin Mueller, John Grabinar

100 Cases in Psychiatry, 2E
Barry Wright, Subodh Dave, Nisha Dogra

100 Cases in Emergency Medicine and Critical Care
Eamon Shamil, Praful Ravi, Dipak Mistry

100 Cases in Clinical Pharmacology, Therapeutics and Prescribing
Kerry Layne, Albert Ferro

100 Cases in Acute Medicine, 2E
Henry Fok, Kerry Layne, Adam Nabeebaccus

100 Cases in Clinical Pathology and Laboratory Medicine, 2E
Eamon Shamil, Praful Ravi, Ashish Chandra

100 Diagnostic Dilemmas in Clinical Medicine, 2E
Kerry Layne

100 Cases in Obstetrics and Gynaecology, 3E
Cecilia Bottomley, Ruth MacSwan, Janice Rymer

For more information about this series please visit: https://www.routledge.com/100-Cases/book-series/CRCONEHUNCAS

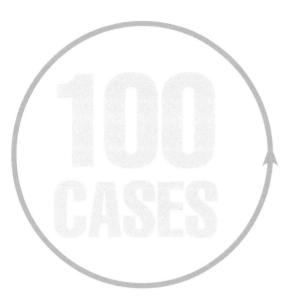

Third Edition

in
Obstetrics and Gynaecology

Cecilia Bottomley MBBChir MRCOG MD
Consultant Gynaecologist
and Honorary Associate Professor
University College London Hospitals (UCLH)
London, UK

Ruth MacSwan
ST6 in Obstetrics and Gynaecology
and Clinical Fellow in Obstetric Ultrasound
University College London Hospitals (UCLH)
London, UK

Janice Rymer MD FRCOG FRANZCOG FHEA
Dean of Student Affairs
and Professor of Obstetrics and Gynaecology
King's College School of Medicine
and Consultant Gynaecologist
Guy's and St Thomas' NHS Foundation Trust
London, UK

100 Cases Series Editor
Janice Rymer

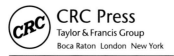

CRC Press
Taylor & Francis Group
Boca Raton London New York

CRC Press is an imprint of the
Taylor & Francis Group, an **informa** business

Third edition published 2025
by CRC Press
2385 NW Executive Center Drive, Suite 320, Boca Raton, FL 33431

and by CRC Press
4 Park Square, Milton Park, Abingdon, Oxon, OX14 4RN

CRC Press is an imprint of Taylor & Francis Group, LLC

© 2025 Cecilia Bottomley, Ruth Macswan and Janice Rymer

This book contains information obtained from authentic and highly regarded sources. While all reasonable efforts have been made to publish reliable data and information, neither the author[s] nor the publisher can accept any legal responsibility or liability for any errors or omissions that may be made. The publishers wish to make clear that any views or opinions expressed in this book by individual editors, authors or contributors are personal to them and do not necessarily reflect the views/opinions of the publishers. The information or guidance contained in this book is intended for use by medical, scientific or health-care professionals and is provided strictly as a supplement to the medical or other professional's own judgement, their knowledge of the patient's medical history, relevant manufacturer's instructions and the appropriate best practice guidelines. Because of the rapid advances in medical science, any information or advice on dosages, procedures or diagnoses should be independently verified. The reader is strongly urged to consult the relevant national drug formulary and the drug companies' and device or material manufacturers' printed instructions, and their websites, before administering or utilizing any of the drugs, devices or materials mentioned in this book. This book does not indicate whether a particular treatment is appropriate or suitable for a particular individual. Ultimately it is the sole responsibility of the medical professional to make his or her own professional judgements, so as to advise and treat patients appropriately. The authors and publishers have also attempted to trace the copyright holders of all material reproduced in this publication and apologize to copyright holders if permission to publish in this form has not been obtained. If any copyright material has not been acknowledged please write and let us know so we may rectify in any future reprint.

ISBN: 9781032480077 (hbk)
ISBN: 9781032397733 (pbk)
ISBN: 9781003386933 (ebk)

DOI: 10.1201/9781003386933

Typeset in Baskerville
by Deanta Global Publishing Services, Chennai, India

Access the Support Material: www.routledge.com/9781032397733

CONTENTS

Section 1: General Gynaecology

Section 2: Emergency Gynaecology

Section 3: Early Pregnancy

Section 4: General Obstetrics

Section 5: Peripartum Care and Obstetric Emergencies

Section 6: Family Planning and Sexual Health

Bonus cases are available for download at www.routledge.com/9781032397733

PREFACE TO THE THIRD EDITION

This book is now in its third edition, a testimony to the popularity of the 100 Cases Series, and the Obstetrics and Gynaecology edition, as a teaching and learning tool.

Reflecting the most up-to-date practice, this edition contains several new cases to reflect contemporary diagnostic and therapeutic tools, while retaining the cases reported to be most useful. The authors are established teachers of undergraduate and postgraduate obstetrics and gynaecology, working daily with and thoroughly understanding the learning needs of medical students and junior doctors in the field.

Real clinical scenarios, from which these cases originate, remain the best way to stimulate thought and understand clinical and pathological processes. Through our question and answer format, the reader is encouraged to practice the skill of formulating investigation and treatment plans as they would in everyday practice.

In this edition we have developed several areas further which reflect the changing landscape of the field, such as pregnancy in the older woman and the management of complex maternal medical conditions in pregnancy.

Engagement of women with the informed consent process and communication skills in general, which are covered extensively, are vitally important in clinical exams.

We have ensured that all of the cases incorporate published national guidance from national bodies such as the National Institute for Health and Care Excellence (NICE) and the Royal College of Obstetricians and Gynaecologists (RCOG) or from specialist societies such as the British Society of Colposcopy and Cervical Pathology (BSCCP).

As with earlier editions, the book is written with both medical students and junior clinicians in their obstetrics and gynaecology placements in mind and has been found to be an ideal tool for both.

Our experience has found that there are always moments in the day between theatre cases, while considering a patient just seen in clinic or after taking a patient history in the emergency department when the cases are pertinent. The simple indexing system means it is easy to find a case to refer to that relates to your current patient, whether that be bleeding in early pregnancy, fibroid management, reduced fetal movements or a postnatal pyrexia.

The cases vary in complexity to reinforce important or common subject areas. The book should reinforce knowledge and build confidence in some areas, challenge and stimulate thought in others and continue to provide an invaluable tool for learning in the specialty of obstetrics and gynaecology.

Cecilia Bottomley
Ruth MacSwan
Janice Rymer

ACKNOWLEDGEMENTS

The authors would like to acknowledge and thank their colleagues for their help with illustrations and useful suggestions for cases for the first, second and third editions of this book.

Section 1
GENERAL GYNAECOLOGY

CASE 1: INTERMENSTRUAL BLEEDING

History

A 48-year-old woman presents with intermenstrual bleeding for 2 months. Episodes of bleeding occur any time in the cycle. This is usually fresh red blood and much lighter than a normal period. It can last for 1–6 days. There is no associated pain. She has no hot flushes or night sweats. She is sexually active and has not noticed vaginal dryness.

She has three children and has used the progesterone-only pill for contraception for 5 years.

Her last smear test was 2 years ago and all smears have been normal. She takes no medication and has no other relevant medical history.

Examination

The abdominal examination is unremarkable. Speculum examination shows a slightly atrophic-looking vagina and cervix but there are no apparent cervical lesions and there is no current bleeding.

On bimanual examination the uterus is non-tender and of normal size, axial and mobile. There are no palpable adnexal masses.

🔍 INVESTIGATIONS

		Normal Range
Haemoglobin	127 g/L	117–157 g/L
White cell count	4.5 × 10⁹/L	3.5–11 × 10⁹/L
Platelets	401 × 10⁹/L	150–440 × 10⁹/L

Transvaginal ultrasound scan and hydrosonography are shown in Figure 1.1.

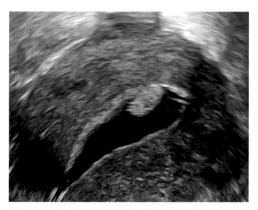

Figure 1.1 Transvaginal ultrasound image showing midsagittal view of the uterine cavity after installation of saline (hydrosonography).

❓ QUESTIONS

- What is the diagnosis and differential diagnosis?
- How would you further investigate and manage this woman?

DOI: 10.1201/9781003386933-2

ANSWER 1

The diagnosis is of an endometrial polyp, shown in the ultrasound image as a mass, surrounded by the instilled fluid, within the endometrial cavity (Figure 1.1). These can occur in women of any age, although they are more common in older women and may be asymptomatic or cause irregular bleeding or discharge. The aetiology is uncertain and the vast majority are benign. In this specific case all the differential diagnoses are effectively excluded by the history and examination.

> **!   DIFFERENTIAL DIAGNOSIS FOR INTERMENSTRUAL BLEEDING**
>
> - Cervical malignancy
> - Cervical ectropion
> - Endocervical polyp
> - Atrophic vaginitis
> - Pregnancy
> - Irregular bleeding related to the contraceptive pill
> - Pelvic inflammatory disease

Management

Any woman should be investigated if bleeding occurs between periods over three cycles or more. In women over the age of 40 years, serious pathology, in particular endometrial carcinoma, should be excluded.

Asymptomatic polyps are common and generally safe to manage expectantly if they demonstrate benign features on ultrasound scan (single feeder vessel, smooth walls, normal surrounding endometrium).

In this case, however, the polyp needs to be removed to eliminate the cause of the bleeding.

Management involves outpatient or day case hysteroscopy, and resection of the polyp under direct vision using a diathermy loop or other resection technique (Figure 1.2). This allows certainty that the polyp had been completely excised and also allows full inspection of the rest of the cavity to check for any other lesions or suspicious areas. In some settings, where hysteroscopic facilities are not available, a dilatation and curettage may be carried out with blind avulsion of the polyp with polyp forceps. This was the standard management in the past but is not the gold standard now, for the reasons explained.

The polyp should be sent for histological analysis to confirm its benign nature.

>   **KEY POINTS**
>
> - Any woman over the age of 40 years should be investigated if bleeding occurs between the periods for more than three cycles, to exclude serious pathology, in particular endometrial carcinoma.
> - Hysteroscopy is rarely indicated for women under the age of 40 years unless pathology is suspected from an ultrasound scan.

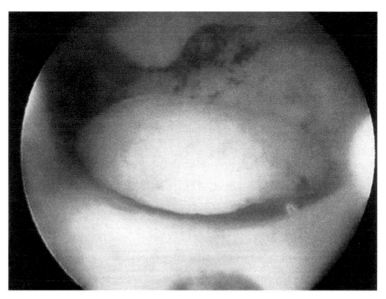

Figure 1.2 Hysteroscopic appearance of endometrial polyp prior to resection.

CASE 2: INFERTILITY

History

A 31-year-old woman has been trying to conceive for nearly 3 years without success. Her last period started 7 months ago and she has been having periods sporadically for about 5 years. She bleeds for 2–7 days and the periods occur at intervals of 2–9 months. There is no dysmenorrhoea but occasionally the bleeding is heavy.

She has been pregnant once in the past at the age of 19 years but that pregnancy was terminated for personal reasons. She had a laparoscopy several years ago for pelvic pain, which showed a normal pelvis.

Cervical smears have always been normal and there is no history of sexually transmitted infection.

The woman was diagnosed with irritable bowel syndrome when she was 25, after thorough investigation for other bowel conditions. She currently uses metoclopramide to increase gut motility, and antispasmodics.

Her partner is fit and well, and has two children by a previous relationship. Neither partner drinks alcohol or smokes.

INVESTIGATIONS

		Normal Range
Follicle-stimulating hormone	3.1 IU/L	Day 2–5 1–11 IU/L
Luteinizing hormone	2.9 IU/L	Day 2–5 0.5–14.5 IU/L
Prolactin	1274 mu/L	90–520 mu/L
Testosterone	1.4 nmol/L	0.8–3.1 nmol/L
Thyroid-stimulating hormone	4.1 mu/L	0.5–7 mu/L
Free thyroxine	17 pmol/L	11–23 pmol/L

Day 21 progesterone was requested but no period occurred for 3 months and therefore the test was not performed.

QUESTIONS

- What is the diagnosis and its aetiology?
- How would you further investigate and manage this couple?

ANSWER 2

The infertility is likely to be secondary to anovulation. Normal testosterone and gonadotrophins and high prolactin suggest the likely case of the anovulation to be hyperprolactinaemia. Hyperprolactinaemia may be physiological in breast-feeding, pregnancy and stress. The commonest causes of pathological hyperprolactinaemia are tumours and idiopathic hypersecretion, but it may also be due to drugs, hypothyroidism, ectopic prolactin secretion or chronic renal failure. In this case the metoclopramide is the cause, as it is a dopamine antagonist (dopamine usually acts via the hypothalamus to cause inhibition of prolactin secretion, and if this is interrupted, prolactin is secreted to excess). Galactorrhoea is not a common symptom of hyperprolactinaemia, occurring in less than half of affected women.

> **!** **DRUGS ASSOCIATED WITH HYPERPROLACTINAEMIA (DUE TO DOPAMINE ANTAGONIST EFFECTS)**
>
> * Metoclopramide
> * Phenothiazines (e.g. chlorpromazine, prochlorperazine, thioridazine)
> * Reserpine
> * Methyldopa
> * Omeprazole, ranitidine, bendrofluazide (rare associations)

The metoclopramide should be stopped and the woman reviewed after 4–6 weeks to ensure that the periods have restarted and that the prolactin level has returned to normal. It would be advisable also at that stage to carry out a day 21 progesterone level to confirm ovulatory cycles.

If the cycles do not resume or the prolactin level does not normalize, then further investigation is needed to exclude other causes of hyperprolactinaemia, such as a pituitary micro- or macroadenoma.

As with all women attempting to conceive, she should have her rubella immunity checked and should be advised to take periconceptual folic acid until 12 weeks of pregnancy to reduce the risk of neural tube defects. She should also be encouraged to be up to date with her COVID and flu immunizations.

If the woman fails to conceive after correction of hyperprolactinaemia, then a full fertility investigation should be planned with semen analysis and tubal patency testing (laparoscopy and dye test, hysterosalpingogram or hysterosalpingo-constrast sonography [HyCoSy]).

> **🔑 KEY POINTS**
>
> * A full drug history should be elicited in women with amenorrhoea or infertility.
> * Galactorrhoea occurs in less than half of women with hyperprolactinaemia.
> * Day 21 progesterone over 30 nmol/L is suggestive of ovulation.

CASE 3: AMENORRHOEA

History

A 32-year-old woman complains that she has not had a period for 3 months. Four home pregnancy tests have all been negative. She started her periods at the age of 15 years and until 30 years she had a normal 27-day cycle. She had one daughter by normal delivery 2 years ago, following which she breast-fed for 6 months. After that she had normal cycles again for several months and then her periods stopped abruptly. She was using the progesterone-only pill for contraception while she was breast-feeding and stopped 6 months ago as she is keen to have another child. She reports symptoms of dryness during intercourse and has experienced sweating episodes at night as well as episodes of feeling extremely hot at any time of day. There is no relevant gynaecological history. The only medical history of note is that she has been hypothyroid for 10 years and takes thyroxine100 mcg per day. She does not take any alcohol, smoke or use recreational drugs.

Examination

Examination findings are unremarkable.

INVESTIGATIONS

		Normal Range
Haemoglobin	122 g/L	117–157 g/L
White cell count	5.1 × 10⁹/L	3.5–11 × 10⁹/L
Platelets	203 × 10⁹/L	150–440 × 10⁹/L
Thyroid-stimulating hormone	3.6 mu/L	0.5–7 mu/L
Free thyroxine	21 pmol/L	11–23 pmol/L
Follicle-stimulating hormone	45 IU/L	Day 2–5 1–11 IU/L
Luteinizing hormone	30 IU/L	Day 2–5 0.5–14.5 IU/L
Prolactin	401 mu/L	90–520 mu/L
Oestradiol	87 pmol/L	Day 2–5 70–510 pmol/L
Testosterone	2.3 nmol/L	0.8–3.1 nmol/L

QUESTIONS

- What is the diagnosis?
- What further investigations should be performed?
- What are the key points in the management of this woman?

DOI: 10.1201/9781003386933-4

ANSWER 3

This woman has symptoms of amenorrhoea as well as hypo-oestrogenic vasomotor symptoms and vaginal dryness. The diagnosis is of premature ovarian insufficiency, confirmed by the very high gonadotrophin levels. High levels occur because the ovary is resistant to the effects of gonadotrophins, and negative feedback to the hypothalamus and pituitary causes increasing secretion to try to stimulate the ovary. Sheehan's syndrome (pituitary necrosis after postpartum haemorrhage) would also cause amenorrhoea but would have inhibited breast-feeding and all menstruation since delivery.

Premature ovarian failure (before the age of 40 years) occurs in 1 per cent of women and has significant physical and psychological consequences. It may be idiopathic but a familial tendency is common. In some cases it is an autoimmune condition (associated with hypothyroidism in this case). Disorders of the X chromosome can also be associated.

> **!　EFFECTS OF PREMATURE MENOPAUSE**
>
> - *Hypo-oestrogenic effects:*
>   - Vaginal dryness
>   - Vasomotor symptoms (hot flushes, night sweats)
>   - Osteoporosis
>   - Increased cardiovascular risk
> - *Psychological and social effects:*
>   - Infertility
>   - Feeling of inadequacy as a woman
>   - Feelings of premature ageing and need to take HRT
>   - Impact on relationships

Further Investigation

Osteoporosis may be prevented with continuous oestrogen replacement, but progesterone should also be given simultaneously (cyclically or continuously) to prevent the increased risk of endometrial carcinoma from unopposed oestrogen. Bone scan is necessary for baseline bone density and to help in monitoring the effects of hormone replacement. Chromosomal analysis and Fragile X-premutation testing is recommended for any woman experiencing premature ovarian insufficiency to identify rare cases due to fragile X syndrome or Turner's syndrome mosaicism. An autoimmune screen should be performed.

Management

Osteoporosis may be prevented with oestrogen replacement, with progesterone protection of the uterus. Traditional HRT preparations or the combined oral contraceptive pill continuously are effective. In terms of future fertility, this woman's options are *in vitro* fertilization (IVF) with donor oocytes, adoption or the acceptance of only having one child. Occasionally, premature ovarian failure is a fluctuating condition (resistant ovary syndrome) whereby the ovaries may function intermittently. Contraception should therefore be used if it would be undesirable to become pregnant. Patient support organizations are a good source for women experiencing such an unexpected and stigmatizing diagnosis.

> 　**KEY POINTS**
>
> - Premature ovarian failure (<40 years) occurs in 1 per cent of women.
> - Oestrogen replacement is essential for bone and cardiovascular protection.
> - It may be possible to conceive with IVF using donor oocytes.

CASE 4: PRIMARY INFERTILITY

History

A couple attends the gynaecology clinic because of failure to conceive. They stopped using condoms for contraception 19 months ago. There are no apparent sexual difficulties, and they have been having intercourse two to three times per week. In the last 6 months, ovulation has been confirmed by the woman reporting a positive home urinary ovulation kit test, and they have been having intercourse around this time.

The woman is 28 years old, with regular 29-day menstrual cycles and no previous gynaecological problems. Both the woman and her partner are generally healthy and have been together for 7 years. Neither reports any previous sexually transmitted infection.

Examination

The woman's investigations are normal, with normal gonadotrophins (LH and FSH), and confirmation of ovulation with a day 21 progesterone test. Chlamydia test is negative and she is immune to rubella. Hysterosalpingogram confirms patent fallopian tubes and normal morphology of the endometrial cavity.

🔍 INVESTIGATIONS

The semen analysis for her partner is as follows:

Parameter		Normal Range (World Health Organization)
Semen volume	3.2 mL	>1.5 mL
Total sperm number	9.6 million	39 million per ejaculate
Sperm concentration	3 million/mL	>15 million/mL
Total motility (progressive and non-progressive)	9%	>40%
Live spermatozoa	45%	>58%
Sperm morphology (normal forms)	3%	>4%

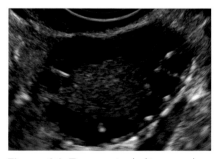

Figure 4.1 Transvaginal ultrasound scan of the ovary.

? QUESTIONS

- What does the semen analysis show?
- What further information should you ascertain from the man?
- What does the ultrasound show and what is its significance in this case?
- What further investigation and management would you plan for the management of this couple's infertility?

DOI: 10.1201/9781003386933-5

ANSWER 4

Semen Analysis Interpretation

Normal ranges for semen characteristics are published by the World Health Organization (WHO). The nomenclature applied to abnormal semen quality depends on the degree of abnormality and the specific type of abnormality. In this case the sample would suggest oligoasthenoterato-zoospermia (total number and concentration of spermatozoa, and percentages of both progressively motile and morphologically normal spermatozoa, all below the lower reference limits).

Further Information to Be Ascertained

The history from the man is insufficient. Further enquiries should include:

- Occupation (infertility has been associated with occupational exposure to chemicals and with scrotal temperature)
- Smoking history
- Alcohol intake
- Previous medical history (cancer treatment, cystic fibrosis, mumps or testicular torsion may affect fertility)
- Medication use (in particular anabolic steroid use as affects spermatogenesis)
- Recent viral illness (may also affect spermatogenesis)

It should be confirmed that the semen sample was provided following the recommended procedures:

- Collected after at least 48 h but no more than 7 days of sexual abstinence
- Delivered to the laboratory within 1 h of production
- Collected by masturbation and ejaculated into a clean glass or plastic container, protected from extremes of temperature (below 20 degrees or above 40 degrees)

Ultrasound Findings

The image shows an ovary which is polycystic in morphology. This is not a relevant factor for this couple as she has regular periods and the day 21 blood test confirms ovulation.

Further Investigation and Management

The abnormal sperm quality is the likely cause of infertility, but the semen analysis must be repeated to confirm that it is not a transient effect, e.g. of a recent viral illness. Causes of oligospermia may be pretesticular (such as pituitary tumours, smoking or medication), testicular (such as varicocoele, trauma, mumps or Y chromosome deletions) or post-testicular (such as prostatitis or cystic fibrosis causing vas deferens obstruction). Referral to an andrologist can be useful in these cases as some causes of oligospermia are amenable to treatment.

The man should also be examined for scrotal size and morphology. Testicular biopsy may be indicated to rule out pathology. Percutaneous sperm aspiration from the testis can be carried out in a man with complete azoospermia from an obstructive cause (not relevant for this couple where the man does have some sperm in the seminal fluid).

Assuming the semen quality remains poor on repeat analysis after 3 months, then the couple will need assisted conception with *in vitro* fertilization and intracytoplasmic sperm injection (direct injection of a single sperm into an egg) to achieve a pregnancy.

CASE 5: INFERTILITY

History

A 37-year-old woman is seen in the clinic because of infertility. She is gravida 2 para 1 having had a daughter 13 years ago, and a miscarriage 2 years later. She separated from her former husband and has now married again and is keen to conceive, especially as her new partner has no children.

Her last period started 45 days ago. She says that her periods are sometimes regular but at other times she has missed a period for up to 3 months. The bleeding is moderate and lasts for up to 4 days. There is no history of pelvic pain or dyspareunia, and no irregular bleeding or discharge. Alcohol intake is minimal and she does not smoke or take other drugs. There is no medical history of note and she takes no regular medication.

Her partner is 34 years old and is also fit and healthy with no significant history of ill-health or medications.

Examination

There are no abnormal features on examination of either partner.

🔍 **INVESTIGATIONS (DURING THE NEXT MENSTRUAL CYCLE)**

		Normal Range
Day 3 follicle-stimulating hormone (FSH)	11.1 IU/L	Day 2–5 1–11 IU/L
Day 3 luteinizing hormone	6.8 IU/L	Day 2–5 0.5–14.5 IU/L
Prolactin	305 mu/L	90–520 mu/L
Testosterone	1.3 nmol/L	0.8–3.1 nmol/L
Day 21 progesterone	13 nmol/L	

Semen analysis report: Normal volume, count, normal forms and motility.
Hysterosalpingogram report: The uterine cavity is of normal shape with a smooth regular outline. Contrast medium is seen to fill both uterine tubes symmetrically and free spill of dye is confirmed bilaterally.
Transvaginal ultrasound scan report: The uterus is anteverted with no congenital abnormalities, uterine fibroids or polyps visualized. Both ovaries are of normal morphology, volume and mobility. Two follicles are seen on the left ovary and one follicle is present on the right ovary.

❓ **QUESTIONS**

- What is the cause of the infertility?
- What are the further investigation and management options?

DOI: 10.1201/9781003386933-6

ANSWER 5

Women with irregular periods often do not ovulate. Anovulation in this case is confirmed by the low day 21 progesterone level. The commonest cause of anovulation is polycystic ovaries, but in this case the ovaries show normal morphology and the androgen levels are normal.

The noticeable abnormality is the high FSH level and the fact that only a small number of follicles are visualized at ultrasound scan. This is suggestive of anovulation from premature failure of ovarian function. The woman is not menopausal because she still has periods, although irregular, and the FSH is only marginally raised. However, it is known that FSH levels above 10 IU/L are associated with a poor prognosis for conception using the woman's own ova.

Further Investigation

The FSH should be repeated, as it is possible that this could be a sporadic result or poorly timed sample, and therefore confirmation is needed before continuing on to treatment.

Anti-Mullerian hormone (AMH) is a further test of ovarian reserve and ovarian responsiveness in women with infertility. It decreases with number of ovarian antral follicles and it can be used to predict likelihood of ovarian response and pregnancy with assisted conception. Optimal fertility is associated with AMH levels of 28–48 pmol/L, whereas levels less than 5 pmol/L are suggestive of poor success rates with natural or assisted conception.

Management

As there is such a poor prognosis for conception either naturally or with *in vitro* fertilization using the woman's own oocytes, she should be counselled about assisted conception using donor eggs. Donated oocytes are fertilized with the partner's sperm and then implanted into the uterus. The woman needs appropriate luteal phase support, most commonly with progesterone pessaries.

!   COUNSELLING ISSUES FOR THIS COUPLE

- *Psychological*:
  - The woman may feel that her ovaries are 'ageing' prematurely and this may have an effect on her self-esteem and sexuality.
  - The stress associated with assisted conception is significant and many couples find that this in itself puts a large burden on their relationship.
- *Funding*: Public funding may not be available as the woman already has one child.
- *Consideration of alternative options*: Adoption, surrogacy and acceptance of not being able to have a child together should be explored with the couple.

   KEY POINTS

- FSH above 10 IU/L is associated with poor prognosis for fertility.
- Infertile couples should be encouraged to explore all options, including accepting childlessness and adoption as well as assisted conception techniques.
- Low AMH is associated with poor fertility. Values less than 5 pmol/L are associated with a very poor chance of IVF success.

CASE 6: SHORTNESS OF BREATH AND ABDOMINAL PAIN

History

A 72-year-old woman has been admitted with shortness of breath. On further questioning she says that she has been unwell for about 8 weeks. She has decreased appetite and nausea when she eats. She has lost weight but her abdomen feels swollen. She has generalized dull abdominal pain and constipation, which is unusual for her. There are no urinary symptoms.

She has always been healthy with no previous hospital admissions. She is a widow and did not have any children. Her periods stopped at 52 years and she has had no postmenopausal bleeding. She has never taken hormone replacement therapy.

Examination

She appears pale and breathless on talking. Chest expansion is reduced on the right side, with dullness to percussion and decreased air entry at the right base. The abdomen is generally distended with shifting dullness. There is a palpable mass which seems to be arising from the pelvis. Speculum examination is normal, but on bimanual palpation there is a fixed left iliac fossa mass of about 10 cm diameter.

INVESTIGATIONS

		Normal Range
Haemoglobin	92 g/L	117–157 g/L
Mean cell volume	82 fL	80–99 fL
White cell count	4.1×10^9/L	$3.5–11 \times 10^9$/L
Platelets	197×10^9/L	$150–440 \times 10^9$/L
Sodium	135 mmol/L	135–145 mmol/L
Potassium	4.0 mmol/L	3.5–5 mmol/L
Urea	5.1 mmol/L	2.5–6.7 mmol/L
Creatinine	89 mmol/L	70–120 mmol/L
Alanine transaminase	18 IU/L	5–35 IU/L
Aspartate transaminase	17 IU/L	5–35 IU/L
Alkaline phosphatase	78 IU/L	30–300 IU/L
Bilirubin	12 mmol/L	3–17 mmol/L
Albumin	30 g/L	35–50 g/L
CA-125	118 ku/L	<30 ku/L

Chest X-ray and abdominal computerized tomography (CT) scan are shown in Figures 6.1 and 6.2, respectively.

? QUESTIONS

- What is the likely diagnosis?
- How should this woman be further investigated?
- If the diagnosis is confirmed how should she be managed?

DOI: 10.1201/9781003386933-7

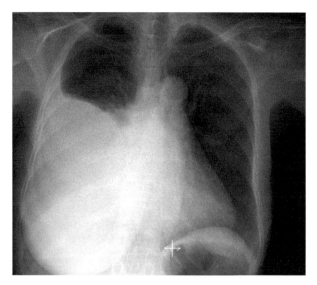

Figure 6.1 Chest X-ray.

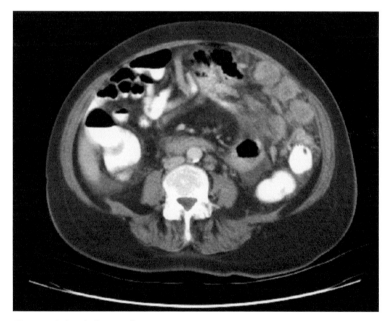

Figure 6.2 Abdominal CT scan.

ANSWER 6

The history and examination are suggestive of a right pleural effusion and ascites. The presence of a pelvic mass would suggest that this is due to an ovarian or bowel problem. The chest X-ray confirms the effusion, and the CT shows a left-sided pelvic tumour and ascites. There are also solid areas in the anterior abdominal wall that represent omental infiltration by the tumour.

CA-125 is a non-specific marker for ovarian carcinoma. The diagnosis is therefore likely to be that of ovarian cancer which commonly presents with systemic symptoms when metastatic disease is already evident.

> ### ! CONFIRMATION OF THE DIAGNOSIS AND MANAGEMENT
>
> The surgical aphorism 'there is no diagnosis without a surgical diagnosis' means that tissue needs to be obtained to confirm the diagnosis. As the suspected tumour has already spread beyond the ovaries, then biopsy does not risk spread of disease and should be performed under radiological guidance, targeting any of the tumour deposits. Where not possible, laparotomy should be performed with three objectives:
>
> 1. Obtaining tissue for diagnosis.
> 2. Staging the disease according to the extent of tissue involvement.
> 3. Primary debulking – to perform a total abdominal hysterectomy and bilateral salping-oophorectomy and to reduce all abdominal tumour deposits to a volume of less than 2 cm. This allows optimal effect of chemotherapy following surgery. Lymph node dissection and omental resection are usually part of the procedure.

Prior to any treatment this woman also needs drainage of her pleural effusion for symptomatic relief and optimization for anaesthetic. She will need referral to her local multidisciplinary gynae oncology team which consists of gynaecologists, oncologists, radiologists, cancer specialist nurses and pathologists. Any extensive operating will be carried out in a large tertiary unit.

The prognosis for ovarian cancer is poor, as most women present at stage 3 or 4.

> ### ! OVARIAN CANCER STAGING AND PROGNOSIS
>
> | Stage | | | Prognosis (5-Year Survival Rate) |
> |---|---|---|---|
> | Stage 1 Confined to the ovaries | 1A | One ovary affected, ovarian capsule is intact | 90% |
> | | 1B | Both ovaries affected, ovarian capsules intact | |
> | | 1C | Ovarian capsule is ruptured, tumour on ovarian surface or malignant cells detected in ascites or peritoneal washings | |
> | Stage 2 Pelvic spread | 2A | Extension or implantation into the uterus and/or fallopian tubes (no malignant cells in ascites/peritoneal washings) | 65% |
> | | 2B | Extension to another organ in the pelvis (no malignant cells in ascites/peritoneal washings) | |
> | | 2C | As for 2A/B plus malignant cells in ascites/peritoneal washings | |

Stage			Prognosis (5-Year Survival Rate)
Stage 3 Peritoneal metastasis outside the pelvis and/or regional lymph node metastasis (includes liver capsule metastasis)	3A	Microscopic peritoneal metastasis beyond the pelvis	35%
	3B	Macroscopic peritoneal metastasis beyond the pelvis (max. diameter 2 cm)	
	3C	Macroscopic peritoneal metastasis beyond the pelvis (max. diameter >2 cm) and/or distant lymph node metastases	
Stage 4 Distant metastasis beyond the peritoneal cavity (or liver parenchymal metastasis)			20%

 KEY POINTS

- CA-125 is a non-specific marker for ovarian cancer.
- Ovarian cancer commonly presents late (stage 3/4) and prognosis is poor.
- Staging and primary treatment is by laparotomy, total abdominal hysterectomy, bilateral salpingoophorectomy and debulking.
- Neoadjuvant chemotherapy (preoperative chemotherapy to shrink the tumour mass down so that debulking surgery is more likely to be successful) may also be considered depending on the extent of disease on imaging.
- Chemotherapy is often effective adjuvant therapy.

CASE 7: ABDOMINAL SWELLING

History

A 36-year-old African-Caribbean woman has noticed abdominal swelling for 10 months. She has to wear larger clothes and people have asked her if she is pregnant, which she finds distressing as she has in fact been trying to conceive. She has no abdominal pain and her bowel habit is normal. She feels nauseated when she eats large amounts. She has urinary frequency but no dysuria or haematuria.

Her periods are regular, every 27 days, and have always been heavy, with clots and flooding on the second and third days. She has never received any treatment for her heavy periods. She has been with her partner for 7 years and despite not using contraception she has never been pregnant.

Examination

The woman has a very distended abdomen. A smooth firm mass is palpable extending from the symphysis pubis to midway between the umbilicus and the xiphisternum (equivalent to a 32-week size pregnancy). It is non-tender and mobile. It is not fluctuant and it is not possible to palpate beneath the mass. On speculum examination it is not possible to visualize the cervix. Bimanual examination reveals a non-tender firm mass occupying the pelvis.

🔎 **INVESTIGATIONS**

		Normal Range
Haemoglobin	63 g/L	117–157 g/L
Mean cell volume	68 fL	80–99 fL
White cell count	4.9×10^9/L	$3.5–11 \times 10^9$/L
Platelets	267×10^9/L	$150–440 \times 10^9$/L

Magnetic resonance images (MRIs) of the abdomen and pelvis are shown in Figures 7.1 and 7.2.

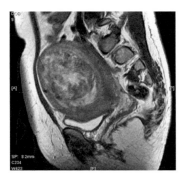

Figure 7.1 MRI of the abdomen and pelvis.

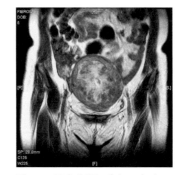

Figure 7.2 MRI of the abdomen and pelvis.

❓ **QUESTIONS**

- What is the diagnosis?
- How would you further investigate and manage this woman?

DOI: 10.1201/9781003386933-8

ANSWER 7

The woman has a large uterine fibroid (leiomyoma). This is causing heavy menstrual bleeding and hence the microcytic anaemia from iron deficiency. Urinary frequency occurs due to the pressure of the large mass on the bladder. It is also possible that the fibroid is contributing to her infertility history, although this warrants investigation as a separate problem.

Fibroids are benign tumours of the myometrium which may be extrinsic (subserous) as in this case. Alternatively, they may be intramural, pedunculated or submucosal (projecting into the endometrial cavity).

! | **TYPICAL PRESENTATIONS OF FIBROIDS**

- Menorrhagia
- Abdominal mass
- Pressure effect from pressure on the bladder, stomach or bowel
- Infertility

Fibroids are not typically painful unless they undergo degeneration (caused by outgrowing their blood supply), usually in pregnancy.

Women of African-Caribbean origin tend to develop fibroids more commonly than women of other ethnic origin.

Further Investigation

Ferritin and folate levels should be checked to confirm the iron-deficiency status. It is also advisable to arrange renal function tests and a renal tract ultrasound, as very large fibroids can cause ureteric obstruction and hydronephrosis, which would need urgent treatment.

Management

The woman should be treated for her anaemia with ferrous sulphate although if very symptomatic may require IV iron preparation (such as ferrinject) or blood transfusion. The heavy menstrual bleeding can be reduced with tranexamic acid during menstruation or she could be offered a levonorgestrel-containing intrauterine device. Gonadotrophin-releasing hormone analogues temporarily shrink fibroids and cause amenorrhoea to allow correction of iron deficiency. Gonadotropin-releasing hormone agonists (GnRHa) are useful in stopping bleeding temporarily to allow anaemia to recover prior to surgery, but are associated with hypoestrogenic side effects such as hot flushes and night sweats. Definitive treatment for fibroids is traditionally by hysterectomy or myomectomy. Myomectomy is favourable for this woman who is keen to have a family, so conservation of the uterus is essential. Uterine artery embolization also causes fibroid degeneration by interruption of the blood supply. However research into long-term safety and potential effects on uterine function during a subsequent pregnancy are not clear.

 | **KEY POINTS**

- Fibroids may be small and incidental or occupy most of the abdomen.
- Anaemia should be suspected in any women with menorrhagia.
- Treatment of fibroids depends on the presence of symptoms, location and the necessity to preserve fertility.
- The optimal operative approach depends on the size and location of the fibroids.

CASE 8: ABNORMAL CERVICAL SMEAR

History

A 28-year-old woman attends the colposcopy clinic after an abnormal liquid-based cytology smear test. She is very anxious as she thinks that she might have cervical cancer. The smear is reported as high-risk (HR) HPV detected and 'severe dyskaryosis'. She had a previous normal (HPV negative) result at age 25 years. She has not had any postcoital or intermenstrual bleeding.

Her first sexual relationship started at the age of 14 years and she has had several partners since then. She lives with her current partner who she has been with for 3 years. She was diagnosed with genital herpes several years ago but has not had any attacks for at least 3 years. She smokes 15–20 cigarettes per day and drinks only at the weekends.

She has an intrauterine contraceptive device *in situ*.

Examination

The cervix is macroscopically normal. At colposcopy, acetic acid is applied and an irregular white area is apparent to the left of the os. Lugol's iodine is applied and the same area stains pale while the rest of the cervix stains dark brown. A biopsy is taken.

🔍 INVESTIGATIONS

Cervical biopsy report: The sample received measures 4 × 2 mm and contains enlarged cells with irregular nuclei consistent with cervical intraepithelial neoplasia 3 (CIN 3).

? QUESTION

- How should this patient be managed?

DOI: 10.1201/9781003386933-9

ANSWER 8

The colposcopy findings show an abnormal area on the left of the cervix. The abnormal tissue stains white with acetic acid because abnormal cells have high-density nuclei which take up the acetic acid more than normal cells. In contrast, abnormal cells have lower glycogen content than normal cells and stain less well, remaining pale when iodine is applied.

The diagnosis is of CIN 3. This is a tissue diagnosis as opposed to dyskaryosis which is an observation of cells from a smear. The degree of dyskaryosis and CIN often correlate, but a dyskaryosis report is not a diagnosis. After a smear showing severe dyskaryosis she has an 80–90 per cent chance of CIN 2 or 3 being found histologically on biopsy at colposcopy.

Management

CIN 3 needs to be treated to prevent progression possibly over several years to cervical carcinoma. The commonest treatment is large-loop excision of the transformation zone (LLETZ) – removal of abnormal cervical tissue with a diathermy loop. Most women tolerate this under local anaesthetic. The LLETZ sample needs to be examined histologically both to confirm removal of all the abnormal tissue, and to ensure that there is not a focus of carcinoma within the sample.

Individuals who have been treated for CIN are at increased risk of developing cervical cancer. A cervical sample should be taken in the community 6 months after treatment. Following that sample:

- All individuals who are negative for HR-HPV are recalled for a repeat cervical sample in a further 3 years.
- All individuals who are positive for HR-HPV must be referred to colposcopy; a reflex cytology sample will be processed to help inform colposcopy.

The woman should be strongly advised to stop smoking as this is a significant modifiable risk factor for the development of cervical carcinoma. Despite exposure to the virus already her risk of future disease is also reduced by the HPV vaccination (if not administered previously).

! ADVICE AFTER LLETZ PROCEDURE

- The patient may have light bleeding for several days.
- If heavy bleeding occurs she should return as secondary infection may occur and need treatment.
- She should avoid sexual intercourse and tampon use for 4 weeks, to allow healing of the cervix.
- Fertility is generally unaffected by the procedure, though cervical stenosis leading to infertility has been reported, and midtrimester loss from cervical weakness is rare.

🔑 KEY POINTS

- Primary high-risk human papilloma virus (HR-HPV) testing is a primary screening tool to identify women at risk of progression to cervical pathology.
- Dyskaryosis refers to an abnormality from a smear.
- Dysplasia and cervical intraepithelial neoplasia are histological terms from a biopsy sample.
- High-grade CIN should be treated to prevent long-term progression to cervical carcinoma.
- HPV vaccination should be advised in women even after prior HPV exposure or infection.

CASE 9: ANAEMIA

History

A 39-year-old woman is referred from the haematologist, with anaemia. She had been complaining of increasing tiredness and shortness of breath for 3 months, with frequent headaches.

Her periods occur every 24 days and the first day is generally moderate but the second to fourth days are very heavy. She uses tampons and sanitary towels together and on the heaviest day she can need to change protection every 30 to 60 minutes. She has no pain. Her last smear test was normal 2 years ago. She has had no previous gynaecological problems and takes no medication.

Examination

The woman is slim with pale conjunctivae. Abdominal, bimanual and speculum examination are unremarkable.

🔍 INVESTIGATIONS

		Normal Range
Haemoglobin	63 g/L	117–157 g/L
Mean cell volume	66 fL	80–99 fL
White cell count	9.1×10^9/L	$3.5–11 \times 10^9$/L
Platelets	300×10^9/L	$150–440 \times 10^9$/L
Ferritin	9 mg/L	6–81 mg/L
Iron	7 mmol/L	10–28 mmol/L
Total iron-binding capacity (TIBC)	80 mmol/L	45–72 mmol/L

Blood film: Hypochromic microcytic red cells.
Transvaginal ultrasound scan report (day 4): The uterus is normal size and retroverted. The endometrium is smooth and thin measuring 3.1 mm. Both ovaries are normal.

❓ QUESTIONS

• How do you interpret these findings?
• What is the likely underlying diagnosis?
• How would you manage this woman?

DOI: 10.1201/9781003386933-10

ANSWER 9

The blood count shows anaemia with reduced mean cell corpuscular volume and low mean cell haemoglobin suggestive of a microcytic anaemia. Iron deficiency is the commonest cause for this picture and is confirmed by the low ferritin and iron, with raised iron-binding capacity. The anaemia accounts for the breathlessness, tiredness and headaches.

Heavy menstrual bleeding is the commonest cause of anaemia in women, and in this case is supported by the history of heavy periods. The woman herself may not recognize that her periods are particularly heavy if she has always experienced heavy periods or if she thinks it is normal for her periods to become heavier as she gets older.

As no other cause of heavy bleeding is apparent from the history and the ultrasound is normal, then the underlying diagnosis is one of exclusion referred to as dysfunctional uterine bleeding (DUB).

Dysfunctional Uterine Bleeding

Excessive heavy, prolonged or frequent bleeding that is not due to pregnancy or any recognizable pelvic or systemic disease.

Management

The anaemia should be treated with ferrous sulphate 200 mg twice daily until haemoglobin and ferritin are normal. It may take 3–6 months for iron stores to be fully replenished. Tranexamic acid (an antifibrinolytic) should be given during menstruation to reduce the amount of bleeding. It is contraindicated with a history of thromboembolic disease. Mefenamic acid (from the non-steroidal anti-inflammatory [NSAID] class of drugs) also helps reduce the blood loss to a lesser extent and these treatments can be used simultaneously.

The levonorgestrel-releasing intrauterine device is used for its action on the endometrium to reduce menorrhagia, often causing amenorrhoea, though it is commonly associated with irregular bleeding for the first 3 months. The combined oral contraceptive pill is effective for menorrhagia in women in whom there are no contraindications.

If these first-line management options are ineffective then endometrial ablation should be considered, which destroys the endometrium down to the basal layer. It is successful in 80–85 per cent of women and they should have completed their family and use effective contraception. There are several approved minimally invasive endometrial ablation techniques with broadly similar efficacy: these include use of radiofrequency waves, electrocautery, microwaves, heated saline or a heated balloon. Amenorrhoea occurs in 30–60 per cent of women with 70–90 per cent describing their satisfaction as good or excellent.

Hysterectomy is considered a 'last resort' for DUB, due to the associated morbidity. If necessary then a total laparoscopic hysterectomy and bilateral salpingectomies with conservation of the ovaries should be offered to minimise the pain and recovery time.

 KEY POINTS

- A woman's perception of bleeding is not always proportionate to the actual volume lost, so haemoglobin should be checked in any woman suspected of menorrhagia.
- DUB is a diagnosis of exclusion.
- A hierarchy of first-, second- and third-line treatment should be used in management.

CASE 10: ABSENT PERIODS

History

A 24-year-old woman presents with the absence of periods for 9 months. She started her periods at the age of 13 years and had a regular 28-day cycle until 18 months ago. The periods then became irregular, occurring every 2–3 months until they stopped completely. She has also had headaches for the last few months and is not sure if this is related. She has a regular sexual partner and uses condoms for contraception. She has never been pregnant. There is no previous medical history of note.

She works as a primary school teacher and drinks approximately 4 units of alcohol per week. She does not smoke or use recreational drugs. She jogs and swims in her spare time.

Examination

The woman is of average build. The blood pressure and general observations are normal. The abdomen is soft and non-tender and speculum and bimanual examination are unremarkable.

INVESTIGATIONS

		Normal Range
Follicle-stimulating hormone	7 IU/L	Day 2–5 1–11 IU/L
Luteinizing hormone	4 IU/L	Day 2–5 0.5–14.5 IU/L
Prolactin	1800 mu/L	90–520 mu/L
Testosterone	1.8 nmol/L	0.8–3.1 nmol/L

Magnetic resonance imaging (MRI) scan of the head is shown in Figure 10.1.

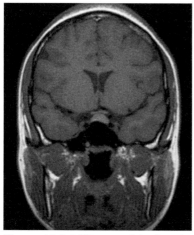

Figure 10.1 MRI scan of the head.

? QUESTIONS

- What is the diagnosis?
- Are any further investigations indicated?
- How would you manage this patient?

DOI: 10.1201/9781003386933-11

ANSWER 10

The investigations show a high-prolactin and a space-occupying lesion in the pituitary fossa in the region of the anterior pituitary as detailed in Figure 10.2. This is consistent with a pituitary adenoma (prolactinoma).

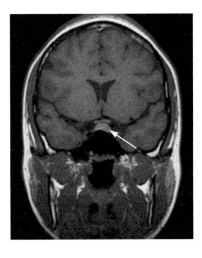

Figure 10.2 Arrow shows a small asymmetrical enlargement of pituitary gland, representative of a small pituitary adenoma (prolactinoma).

Prolactin should always be measured in a woman with amenorrhoea. Care should be taken in interpreting the results, as levels up to 1000 mu/L can be found as a result of stress (even due to venepuncture), breast examination or in association with polycystic ovarian syndrome. Above 1000 mu/L the usual cause is a pituitary adenoma (micro- or macroscopic).

!   **DIFFERENTIAL DIAGNOSIS OF SECONDARY AMENORRHOEA**

- *Hypothalamic*:
  - Chronic illness
  - Anorexia/low BMI
  - Excessive exercise
  - Stress
- *Pituitary*:
  - Hyperprolactinaemia (e.g. drugs, tumour)
  - Hypothyroidism
  - Breast-feeding
- *Ovarian*:
  - Polycystic ovarian insufficiency
  - Premature ovarian failure
  - Iatrogenic (chemotherapy, radiotherapy, oophorectomy)
  - Long-acting progesterone contraception
- *Uterine*:
  - Pregnancy
  - Asherman's syndrome
  - Cervical stenosis

Further Investigation

The visual fields should be checked, as visual field defects may be present with a large tumour. Thyroid function should be tested as hypothyroidism is also a cause of amenorrhoea. The other important investigation in any woman with amenorrhoea is a pregnancy test, although with this history this would be very unlikely. (Prolactin is also raised in pregnancy.)

Management

Most prolactinomas respond to medical treatment with bromocriptine or cabergoline. These are both dopamine agonists, which inhibit prolactin secretion from the anterior pituitary. Cabergoline is generally the first-line agent in the management of prolactinomas and idiopathic hyperprolactinaemia due to higher affinity for D2 receptor sites, more rapid resolution of prolactin levels, menstruation and return of ovulatory cycles and a better side effect profile.

Maintaining the prolactin level below 1000 mu/L causes menstruation (and ovulation) to return in most women. This can be continued indefinitely or until pregnancy is achieved if the presenting complaint is of infertility.

 KEY POINTS

- Hyperprolactinaemia is a common cause of secondary amenorrhoea.
- Prolactin levels up to 1000 u/L may be due to non-pathological causes such as stress.
- Prolactinomas can usually be treated effectively with medical suppression, and surgery is only indicated rarely.

CASE 11: POSTMENOPAUSAL BLEEDING

History

A 59-year-old woman awoke with blood on her nightdress, which was bright red but not heavy. There were no clots of blood and there was no associated pain. The bleeding has recurred twice since in similar amounts.

Her last period was at the age of 49 years and she has had no other intervening bleeding episodes. She suffered hot flushes and night sweats around the time of her menopause, which have now stopped. She is sexually active but has noticed vaginal dryness on intercourse recently.

She has always had normal cervical smears, the last one being 7 months ago. She had two children by spontaneous vaginal delivery and had a laparoscopic sterilization aged 34 years. She has never used hormone replacement therapy (HRT). She takes atenolol for hypertension and omeprazole for epigastric pain.

Examination

The body mass index (BMI) is 28 kg/m². Abdominal examination is normal. The vulva and vagina appear thin and atrophic and the cervix is normal. The uterus is small and anteverted and with no palpable adnexal masses.

An outpatient endometrial biopsy is taken at the time of examination and sent for histological examination.

🔍 INVESTIGATIONS

Transvaginal ultrasound scan is shown in Figure 11.1.

Endometrial biopsy report: The specimen shows atrophic endometrium with no evidence of inflammation, hyperplasia or malignancy.

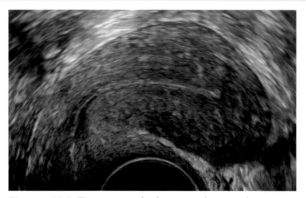

Figure 11.1 Transvaginal ultrasound scan showing a midsagittal view of the uterus and endometrial 'stripe'. The endometrial thickness is measured to be 2.8 mm.

❓ QUESTIONS

- What is the likely diagnosis?
- How would you manage this patient?

DOI: 10.1201/9781003386933-12

ANSWER 11

Postmenopausal bleeding is considered to be caused by endometrial cancer until proven otherwise. However only 10 per cent of women with postmenopausal bleeding are diagnosed with endometrial cancer.

> **! CAUSES OF POSTMENOPAUSAL BLEEDING**
>
> - Endometrial cancer
> - Endometrial/endocervical polyp
> - Endometrial hyperplasia
> - Atrophic vaginitis
> - Iatrogenic (anticoagulants, intrauterine device, hormone replacement therapy)
> - Infective (vaginal candidiasis)

In this case the endometrium is <3 mm on ultrasound, which effectively excludes an endometrial malignancy or polyp. The normal endometrial biopsy report confirms the absence of endometrial pathology. The smear history is normal, and the cervix appears normal, excluding cervical cancer. She is not taking any medication that may predispose to abnormal bleeding.

The diagnosis of atrophic vaginitis can therefore be made by exclusion of serious causes, and is backed up by the history of vaginal dryness at sexual intercourse and the atrophic vulva and vagina noted on examination.

Management

Treatment is hormonal with a course of topical oestrogen given daily for 2 weeks and then twice weekly for maintenance, for an initial period of 2–3 months. An alternative solution is to give a combined form of systemic HRT to protect the endometrium.

Some women are reluctant to use HRT because of the associated risks, and therefore advice should be given about vaginal moisturisers which decrease discomfort but have no reparative value. If bleeding recurs after treatment or the diagnosis is in doubt, then further investigation with hysteroscopy and biopsy, ideally as an outpatient procedure, is needed.

> **🔑 KEY POINTS**
>
> - Women with postmenopausal bleeding (PMB) should be considered to have endometrial cancer until proven otherwise.
> - Endometrial thickness, endometrial biopsy and hysteroscopy are used to investigate PMB.
> - Endometrial thickness less than 4 mm in a woman with postmenopausal bleeding reduces the probability of carcinoma to less than 3 per cent (although individual protocols may use different cutoff levels).
> - Atrophic vaginitis can be treated with courses of topical oestrogens.

CASE 12: PAINFUL PERIODS

History

A 43-year-old woman is referred from her general practitioner (GP) with painful periods. She says that her periods have always been quite heavy and painful but that in the last 2–3 years they have become almost unbearable. She bleeds every 24 days and the period lasts for 7–9 days with very heavy flow from day 2 to day 6. The pain starts approximately 36 h before the onset of the bleeding and lasts until about day 5. The pain is constant, dull and severe, such that she cannot do any housework or any social activities during this time. Her GP has prescribed paracetamol and mefenamic acid in combination, which she says 'takes the edge off' but does not fully relieve the symptoms.

She has had four normal deliveries and her husband had a vasectomy several years ago.

There is no history of intermenstrual or postcoital discharge and she has no abnormal discharge. Her smear history is normal, the most recent being 18 months ago. She takes citalopram for depression but currently reports her mood as fine. She does not drink alcohol or smoke.

Examination

The abdomen is soft and there is vague tenderness in the suprapubic area. The cervix appears normal. On bimanual palpation the uterus is approximately 10 weeks size, soft and bulky. She is tender on palpation but there is no cervical excitation, adnexal tenderness or adnexal masses.

INVESTIGATIONS

Transvaginal ultrasound scan is shown in Figure 12.1.

Transvaginal ultrasound report: There is asymmetrical uterine enlargement, with a thickened posterior uterine wall. There are ill-defined cystic spaces within the myometrium. There is an indistinct myometrial-endometrial border. Both ovaries appear normal in size and morphology.

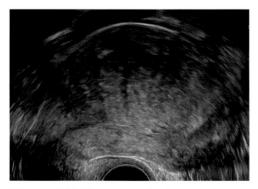

Figure 12.1 Transvaginal ultrasound scan showing a midsagittal view of the uterus.

? QUESTIONS

- What is the likely diagnosis?
- How would you further investigate and manage this woman?

DOI: 10.1201/9781003386933-13

ANSWER 12

The symptoms of dysmenorrhoea and heavy vaginal bleeding along with the ultrasound report suggest a diagnosis of adenomyosis. This is a benign condition whereby functioning endometrial glands and stroma are found within the myometrium. With each period bleeding occurs from the endometrial tissue into the smooth muscle, with associated pain. It tends to occur in women over 35 years and risk factors include increased parity, termination and previous caesarean section. The condition may commonly be found in association with endometriosis. Classically the diagnosis may only be made histologically after hysterectomy for dysmenorrhoea. More recently, however, the diagnosis can be suspected by ultrasound or magnetic resonance imaging (MRI) scan.

! CAUSES OF DYSMENORRHOEA

- Idiopathic
- Premenstrual syndrome
- Pelvic inflammatory disease
- Endometriosis
- Adenomyosis
- Submucosal pedunculated fibroids
- Iatrogenic (e.g. intrauterine contraceptive device [IUCD] or cervical stenosis after large-loop excision of the transformation zone [LLETZ])

Further Investigation

If the diagnosis is in doubt then an MRI scan may be requested, however ultrasonography is becoming more reliable at diagnosing adenomyosis. Hysterectomy to obtain histological diagnosis would be inappropriate.

Management

The initial management is trial of NSAID (unless contraindicated). There is no evidence to recommend mefenamic acid over ibuprofen. Tranexamic acid reduces the amount of bleeding, and this may secondarily reduce the amount of pain. As this patient does not wish to conceive, using hormonal treatment for a 3–6-month trial would be appropriate. This could be in the form of progesterone only pill (POP), combined contraceptive pill (COCP) (which can be run back to back), Depo-Provera injection every 3 months or insertion of a levonorgestrel-releasing intrauterine device. Suppression of menstruation can be achieved with gonadotrophin-releasing hormone analogues however this cannot be used in the long term unless given with add back hormone replacement therapy to reduce the chance of developing osteopenia.

As a last resort hysterectomy should be performed.

🔑 KEY POINTS

- The prevalence of adenomyosis is unknown.
- It is a cause of heavy menstrual bleeding and dysmenorrhoea.
- Hysterectomy may be avoided by use of analgesia or hormonal suppression.

CASE 13: POSTCOITAL BLEEDING

History

An 18-year-old woman is referred with postcoital bleeding. It has occurred on approximately seven occasions over the preceding 6 weeks. Generally it has been a small amount of bright red blood noticed a few hours after intercourse and lasting up to 2 days. There is no associated pain.

Her last period started 3 weeks ago and she bleeds for 4 days every 28 days. Her periods were previously quite heavy but are now lighter since starting the combined oral contraceptive pill (COCP) 6 months ago. There is no history of an abnormal discharge or offensive odour and she has no dyspareunia.

She has had three sexual partners and has been with her current partner for 10 months. She has never been diagnosed with a sexually transmitted infection. She had an appendectomy at the age of 7 years and was diagnosed with epilepsy in childhood but has been off all medication and fit-free for 8 years.

Examination

The abdomen is soft and non-tender. Speculum examination reveals a florid reddened area symmetrically surrounding the external cervical os with contact bleeding. The uterus is normal sized, anteverted and non-tender. There is no cervical excitation and the adnexae are unremarkable.

? | **QUESTIONS**

- What is the differential diagnosis?
- What further investigations would you perform for this woman?
- If your investigations are negative what is the likely diagnosis and how would you manage the woman?

DOI: 10.1201/9781003386933-14

ANSWER 13

Postcoital bleeding in a young woman is common and normally benign. In this specific case the examination findings are consistent only with cervical ectropion, malignancy or infection.

! DIFFERENTIAL DIAGNOSES OF POSTCOITAL BLEEDING IN A YOUNG WOMAN

- Cervical ectropion
- Chlamydia or other sexually transmitted infection (STI)
- Cervical malignancy
- Complication of the COCP
- Endocervical polyp

🔍 INVESTIGATIONS

An STI screen should be performed:

- Endocervical swab for chlamydia
- Endocervical swab for gonorrhoea
- High vaginal swab for trichomonas (and candida, not a STI, but possibly a cause of irregular bleeding from vaginitis)

A cervical smear should also be taken to exclude cervical intraepithelial neoplasia or malignancy prior to treatment.

Management

Assuming the swabs and smear are negative then the diagnosis is of a bleeding cervical ectropion. This is particularly common around the time of puberty, in women using the COCP and in pregnancy. It is not of clinical significance and is generally an incidental finding but warrants treatment if it causes embarrassing and troublesome bleeding (or discharge in some cases).

There are three options for treatment:

1. Stop the COCP and use alternative contraception.
2. Cold coagulation or silver nitrate treatment of the cervix.
3. Diathermy ablation of the ectocervix.

🔑 KEY POINTS

- Cervical ectropion is very common and usually incidental and asymptomatic.
- It occurs particularly in pregnancy and with use of the COCP.
- Postcoital bleeding should always be investigated to exclude significant pathology.

CASE 14: RECURRENT MISCARRIAGE

History

A 34-year-old woman is referred from the emergency department with vaginal bleeding at 6 weeks and 5 days' gestation. Bleeding started 2 days ago initially as 'spotting' but has now increased such that she needs to change a sanitary towel regularly. There is a mild dull lower abdominal pain.

She normally has a regular 28-day cycle. In the past she has used the combined oral contraceptive pill but stopped 3 years ago when she and her partner decided to start a family.

She is gravida 3 para 0. Her first pregnancy ended in a spontaneous complete miscarriage at 6 weeks' gestation 2 years ago. Five months ago she underwent surgical management for an early embryonic demise at 9 weeks' gestation.

There is no gynaecological history of note. Medically she is fit and healthy, except for mild asthma for which she takes inhalers.

The woman's mother died from a pulmonary embolism after her last child. Her brother also had a deep venous thrombosis at the age of 29 years. Her sister has two children, both born preterm because of severe pre-eclampsia.

Examination

The abdomen is non-distended but tender suprapubically. The cervical os is open and products of conception are removed and sent for histological examination.

The bleeding subsequently settles.

🔍 INVESTIGATIONS

		Normal Range for Pregnancy
Haemoglobin	111 g/L	110–140 g/L
White cell count	3.9×10^9/L	6–16 × 10^9/L
Platelets	201×10^9/L	150–400 × 10^9/L

Anticardiolipin antibody: Positive
Lupus anticoagulant: Positive

Histology report: Chorionic villi are seen, confirming products of conception, with no abnormal trophoblast proliferation.

? QUESTIONS

- What is the likely underlying diagnosis for the recurrent miscarriages?
- What further investigation should be performed?
- How should this patient be managed?

DOI: 10.1201/9781003386933-15

ANSWER 14

Raised anticardiolipin antibodies and lupus anticoagulant are suggestive of antiphospholipid syndrome.

! **DIAGNOSIS OF ANTIPHOSPHOLIPID SYNDROME**

- *The presence of one of the clinical features:*
  - Three or more consecutive miscarriages
  - Midtrimester fetal loss
  - Severe early-onset pre-eclampsia, intrauterine growth restriction or abruption
  - Arterial or venous thrombosis
- *And haematological features:*
  - Anticardiolipin antibody or lupus anticoagulant detected on two occasions at least 6 weeks apart

---

Thus in this case the diagnosis must be confirmed by a second positive anticardiolipin test after at least 6 weeks. She should also be tested for antinuclear and anti-double-stranded DNA antibodies as antiphospholipid syndrome may be secondary to systemic lupus erythematosus (SLE).

As this is her third miscarriage it would have been prudent to send the products of conception for karyotyping, as chromosomal abnormalities (typically a balanced translocation) in one parent account for 3–5 per cent of recurrent miscarriages. If a chromosomal abnormality is identified then karyotyping of both partners may be indicated, depending on the specific abnormality.

Management

In the context of antiphospholipid syndrome, oral low-dose aspirin and low-molecular-weight subcutaneous heparin from the time of a positive pregnancy test should be given in subsequent pregnancies to improve the likelihood of a successful live birth.

In the case of this woman, with such a strong family history of thrombosis and proven antiphospholipid syndrome, she would also be recommended thromboprophylaxis throughout the pregnancy and postnatal period with low-molecular-weight heparin, to protect her from venous thromboembolism.

There is no proven benefit from progesterone in women with recurrent miscarriage. Psychological support should be given with regular reassurance ultrasound scans in the first trimester. There is some evidence that shows repeated ultrasound scans for reassurance alone improve the outcome after recurrent miscarriage.

! **CAUSES OF RECURRENT MISCARRIAGE**

- Antiphospholipid syndrome (up to 15 per cent women with recurrent miscarriage)
- Parental chromosome abnormality (3–5 per cent, e.g. balanced translocation)
- Other thrombophilia (e.g. activated protein C resistance)
- Uterine abnormality (intracavity fibroids, uterine septum)
- Uncontrolled diabetes or hypothyroidism
- Bacterial vaginosis (usually associated with second-trimester loss)
- Cervical weakness ('incompetence', second-trimester loss only)

KEY POINTS

- Only a minority of women with recurrent miscarriage will have a cause identified.
- Aspirin and heparin are effective in women with antiphospholipid syndrome.
- Reassurance ultrasound scans and support may improve outcome for women with recurrent loss.

CASE 15: PELVIC PAIN

History

A 29-year-old woman presents with lower abdominal pain for 4 years occurring with her periods. She takes paracetamol and ibuprofen and goes to bed with a hot water bottle for up to 2 days every month. For the last 18 months pain has also occurred between periods.

The pain is dull and constant across the lower abdomen. Her periods are regular and there is no menorrhagia, intermenstrual or postcoital bleeding. There is no other significant medical history.

She has been married for 2 years and has deep dyspareunia which causes interruption of intercourse. She does not use any contraception, as they are keen to start a family. She has never been pregnant in the past.

Examination

There is generalized lower-abdominal tenderness, particularly in the suprapubic area, but no masses are palpable. Speculum examination is unremarkable. On bimanual palpation the uterus is axial and fixed with cervical excitation. The pouch of Douglas is very tender and contains a mass. The adnexae are both tender but no adnexal masses are palpable.

 INVESTIGATIONS

Transvaginal ultrasound scan is shown in Figure 15.1.

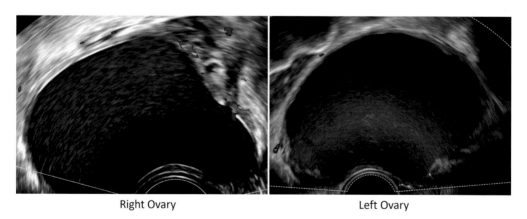

| Right Ovary | Left Ovary |

Figure 15.1 Transvaginal ultrasound scan showing the ovaries in the pouch of Douglas.

? **QUESTIONS**

- What is the diagnosis?
- How would you further manage this woman?

DOI: 10.1201/9781003386933-16

ANSWER 15

The history of dysmenorrhoea and dyspareunia is classic for endometriosis, and the ultrasound examination images show bilateral endometriomas ('chocolate cysts'), a complication of this disease.

Endometriosis is a common condition where active endometrial glands and stroma are located outside the endometrial cavity. Endometriomas develop as ectopic endometrial tissue on the ovary produces blood, which builds up into an encapsulated cyst with each consecutive menstrual cycle.

Endometriosis is benign but carries a high physical and psychological morbidity due to the clinical features:

- Pelvic pain
- Dysmenorrhoea
- Dyspareunia
- Infertility

Examination findings include tenderness or a pelvic mass, and may include palpable nodules in the rectovaginal septum and a fixed retroverted uterus secondary to adhesions (the 'frozen pelvis').

Transvaginal ultrasound features such as these ovarian cysts containing 'ground-glass' echoes can be diagnostic of endometriosis. Other features of moderate or severe endometriosis on ultrasound examination might include visible solid endometriotic nodules within the rectovaginal space or uterosacral ligaments. Superficial endometriosis is often not evident on ultrasound scan however and may only be detected laparoscopically.

Management

Medical suppression of endometriosis is possible with the contraceptive pill or gonadotrophin-releasing hormone analogues (GnRHa), which inhibit ovulation and hence prevent stimulation of endometrial deposits by oestrogen. The levonorgestrel-releasing intrauterine device is also used to suppress endometriosis and reduce symptoms, as do the progesterone-only or combined contraceptive pills.

The mainstay of management for endometriosis has been surgical, with ablation or excision of endometriotic deposits by laparoscopy. In this case there are bilateral endometriotic cysts that need to be removed laparoscopically by cystectomy or just drained. Often pretreatment with GnRHa helps reduce the size of the endometrioma and makes the disease less active before surgery. Surgical treatment should relieve the dyspareunia and dysmenorrhoea at least in the short term and may improve fertility in more severe disease. However studies suggest a decline in ovarian reserve following ovarian endometrioma surgery and so practice now is that surgery should be carried out only after considering carefully the potential benefits and risks.

Consideration should be given to referring to a gynaecologist if in primary care, and preferably a specialist endometriosis service.

!	KEY POINTS

- Endometriosis classically presents with dysmenorrhoea, dyspareunia and infertility.
- Endometriosis is often diagnosed years after symptoms start.
- Surgical excision is required in some cases of severe disease if conservative measures have not been effective.

CASE 16: INFERTILITY

History

A 31-year-old woman and her 34-year-old partner are referred by the general practitioner because of primary infertility. They have been trying to conceive for over 2 years. The woman has regular menstrual periods, bleeding for 4 days every 28–30 days. Her periods are not heavy and have never been painful. There is no intermenstrual bleeding or discharge and no postcoital bleeding. She has never been diagnosed with a sexually transmitted infection.

The last smear was negative 1 year ago. She is a non-smoker and drinks alcohol very occasionally.

The partner's only previous medical history was an appendectomy and a course of anti-*Helicobacter* therapy after he developed epigastric pain and was diagnosed with the infection. He previously smoked 20 cigarettes per day and drank up to 28 units of alcohol per week but has now stopped smoking and significantly reduced his alcohol intake. He works as a buyer for a retail company.

The couple has intercourse 1–4 times per week and there is no reported sexual dysfunction or pain on intercourse. They both deny recreational drug use.

Examination

On examination the woman has a BMI of 23 kg/m². There is no hirsutism or acne. There are no signs of thyroid disease. The abdomen is soft and non-tender. Speculum and bimanual palpation are unremarkable. Genital examination of the partner is also normal.

🔍 INVESTIGATIONS

		Normal Range
Follicle-stimulating hormone (day 3)	4.2 IU/L	Day 2–5 1–11 IU/L
Luteinizing hormone (day 3)	2.7 IU/L	Day 2–5 0.5–14.5 IU/L
Day 21 progesterone	45 nmol/L	
Prolactin	374 mu/L	90–520 mu/L
Testosterone	2.0 nmol/L	0.8–3.1 nmol/L
Semen analysis		
Volume	4 mL	2–5 mL
Count	63 million/mL	>20 million/mL
Normal forms	22 per cent	>15 per cent normal shape
Motility	53 per cent progressively mobile	>50 per cent progressively mobile

Rubella antibody: Immune
Chlamydia: Negative

A hysterosalpingogram is shown in Figure 16.1.

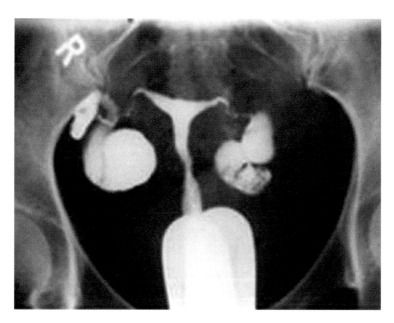

Figure 16.1 Hysterosalpingogram.

ANSWER 16

Day 21 progesterone above 30 nmol/L confirms ovulation, and this is supported by normal follicle-stimulating hormone (FSH), luteinizing hormone (LH) and prolactin. Normal testosterone suggests that polycystic ovaries is an unlikely diagnosis.

The semen analysis is normal, and therefore any male factor aetiology is unlikely. Rubella immunity should always be confirmed.

The hysterosalpingogram shows fill of contrast medium into both uterine tubes (which appear dilated) but no spill, suggesting tubal obstruction as the cause of the fertility problem.

Further Investigation

Tubal blockage on hysterosalpingogram can sometimes be due to tubal spasm, and therefore a laparoscopy and dye may be needed to confirm the pathology and also to determine a cause such as adhesions from previous infection or possibly endometriosis (although the history does not support this diagnosis).

Management

If the tubes are found to be patent, then this would suggest that it is feasible to attempt pregnancy with *in utero* insemination. However, if blocked tubes are confirmed then *in vitro* fertilization (IVF) is indicated. Abnormal tubes are usually removed (or have clips placed across them) prior to IVF, as success rates for pregnancy are better and ectopic pregnancy rate reduced after bilateral salpingectomy.

General advice should be given to take folic acid 400 mg daily to reduce the risk of neural tube defects, and to the partner to minimize his alcohol intake.

In this case a laparoscopy was performed which showed bilateral hydrosalpinges and adhesions as well as perihepatic 'violin-string' adhesions. These findings are consistent with previous infection with chlamydia (or more rarely gonorrhoea). It is not unusual to find such severe pelvic adhesions even when there has never been a clear clinical history of pelvic infection or sexually transmitted infection. Although the infection may be long ago, it is sensible to treat both the woman and her partner with a course of antibiotics for pelvic inflammatory disease.

 KEY POINTS

- Infertility may be due to anovulation, tubal or endometrial/uterine pathology as well as male factors.
- Up to 30 per cent of infertile couples have more than one factor causing infertility.
- Tubal obstruction on hysterosalpingogram is not always confirmed at laparoscopy.

CASE 17: HEAVY MENSTRUAL BLEEDING

History

A 39-year-old woman complains of increasingly long and heavy periods over the last 5 years. Previously she bled for 4 days but now bleeding lasts up to 10 days. The periods still occur every 28 days. She experiences intermenstrual bleeding between most periods but no postcoital bleeding.

The periods were never painful previously but in recent months have become extremely painful with intermittent cramps. She has had four normal deliveries and had a laparoscopic sterilization after her last child. Her smear tests have always been normal, the most recent being 4 months ago. She has never had any previous irregular bleeding or any other gynaecological problems.

Examination

The abdomen is soft and non-tender with no palpable masses. Speculum examination shows a normal cervix. On bimanual palpation the uterus is bulky (approximately 8-week size), mobile and anteverted. There are no adnexal masses.

🔍 INVESTIGATIONS

		Normal Range
Haemoglobin	92 g/L	117–157 g/L
Mean cell volume	75 fL	80–99 fL
White cell count	4.5×10^9/L	$3.5–11 \times 10^9$/L
Platelets	198×10^9/L	$150–440 \times 10^9$/L

Findings at hysteroscopy are shown in Figure 17.1.

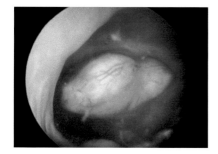

Figure 17.1 Hysteroscopy image.

? QUESTIONS

- What is the diagnosis?
- What further preoperative non-invasive investigation might have allowed the same diagnosis?
- How would you manage this patient and counsel her about the management and its potential risks?

ANSWER 17

The hysteroscopy shows a submucosal fibroid. Ultrasound scan would have provided a preoperative diagnosis too. At hysteroscopy a submucosal fibroid appears as a solid, pale, smooth, relatively immobile (unless pedunculated) structure, whereas a polyp appears pink, fleshy and highly mobile. Submucosal fibroids are a common cause of menorrhagia and can cause, as in this case, intermenstrual bleeding. The cramp-like pain occurs as the uterus tries to expel the fibroid. In some cases this eventually occurs with the fibroid becoming pedunculated and extending through to the vagina on a pedicle. Submucosal fibroids may be also associated with subfertility and require removal prior to fertility treatment.

Management

The management is by hysteroscopic (transcervical) resection of the fibroid (TCRF). This can be performed as a day case under general anaesthetic (or even local anaesthetic if the fibroid is small). The important points in counselling the patient are as follows.

- *Description of the procedure*: The procedure involves stretching (dilatation) of the cervix and insertion of an endoscope into the uterus (hysteroscopy) to view the fibroid. The fibroid is 'shaved' away with a hot wire loop (diathermy). Fluid is circulated through the uterine cavity to enhance the view and allow cooling.
- *What are the risks?*
  - Bleeding: It is rare to bleed heavily but in the unusual extreme situation blood transfusion could be required, and other measures considered to control bleeding such as intracavity balloon placement or uterine artery embolization.
  - Infection: A single dose of prophylactic antibiotic may be administered.
  - Fluid overload: During the procedure, irrigation fluid is absorbed into the circulation. Excessive absorption can cause breathing difficulties (pulmonary oedema) and the need for hospital admission (though this is less common now with the use of modern bipolar devices which use saline rather than glycine).
  - Uterine perforation: Rarely the hysteroscope perforates the wall of the uterus, and if this occurs or is suspected then laparoscopy is needed immediately to confirm it, secure any bleeding and check for damage to surrounding bowel or bladder.
- *What to expect afterwards*: Most women experience bleeding, discharge and passing of 'debris' for 2 to 6 weeks after the procedure.

 KEY POINTS

- Ultrasound is critical in the diagnosis of menorrhagia.
- Submucosal fibroids are more likely to cause menorrhagia than those that are intramural or subserosal.
- Transcervical resection of fibroids is a relatively simple procedure but may be associated with important risks.

CASE 18: URINARY INCONTINENCE

History

A 61-year-old woman complains of involuntary loss of urine. She has noticed it gradually over the last 10 years and has finally decided to see her general practitioner about it after hearing a programme on the radio about treatment for incontinence. The leaking is generally of small amounts and she wears a pad all the time. It tends to occur when she cannot get to the toilet in time. She never leaks on coughing or sneezing. She suffers urgency, particularly when she comes home after being out and is about to come into the house. She also has frequency, passing urine every hour during the day and getting up two or three times each night.

Due to the incontinence she tries not to drink much and usually has two cups of tea first thing in the morning, coffee mid-morning and a further cup of tea mid-afternoon. Other than that she drinks one glass of squash per day and has one glass of wine at night.

She is a non-smoker. She has had two uncomplicated vaginal deliveries. Her periods stopped at the age of 54 years. There is no other gynaecological or medical history of note.

Examination

Abdominal examination is normal. On vaginal examination there is minimal uterovaginal descent and no anterior or posterior vaginal wall prolapse.

 INVESTIGATIONS

Midstream urinalysis: Protein negative, blood negative, leucocytes negative, nitrites negative.

Urodynamics: The first urge to void was reported at 150 mL bladder filling. Involuntary detrusor contractions were noted while the patient was attempting to inhibit micturition. There was no loss of urine with coughing.

? **QUESTIONS**

- What is the diagnosis?
- How would you advise and manage this patient?

DOI: 10.1201/9781003386933-19

ANSWER 18

The diagnosis is of urge urinary incontinence and overactive bladder syndrome (OAB), defined as urgency that occurs with or without urge incontinence (UI) and usually with frequency and nocturia. This was formerly referred to as detrusor instability. In this condition the bladder contracts involuntarily without the normal trigger to void caused by bladder filling. This results in involuntary loss of urine that is embarrassing and often impacts enormously on women's lives, as they are constantly aware of needing to void and where the nearest toilet might be.

Prior to further investigation she should be asked to complete a bladder diary to assess extent of symptoms.

It is important to exclude other causes of such symptoms (such as urinary tract infection or a bladder tumour) with urine microscopy and culture. This should be the first-line investigation in all women with urinary incontinence.

Urodynamic investigation with filling and voiding cystometry is helpful (as in this case) in confirming the diagnosis by showing spontaneous detrusor contractions during bladder filling.

Management

- *Conservative*:
  - The woman should be advised that both caffeine and alcohol are bladder stimulants and are likely to worsen symptoms so should be minimized. She should take a normal fluid intake per day but avoid drinks after about 7 pm to limit nocturia.
  - Bladder retraining for 6 weeks, involving a 'drill' restricting voiding to increasing intervals should be taught.
- *Medical treatment*:
  - If lifestyle advice and bladder retraining fail then anticholinergic medication such as oxybutynin, tolterodine, fesoterodine or darifenacin should be commenced. The associated side effects to be warned of include dry eyes, dry mouth and constipation. Mirabegron is a beta-3-adrenoceptor agonist, which may be used if anticholinergics fail.
  - The effects of treatment should be monitored using one of the validated incontinence-specific quality-of-life scales.

 KEY POINTS

- Overactive bladder syndrome is associated with urgency, frequency and urge incontinence.
- Conservative measures are bladder retraining and caffeine avoidance.
- Medical treatment is generally with anticholinergics.

CASE 19: ABSENT PERIODS

History

An 18-year-old woman presents with an absence of periods for 6 months. This has occurred twice before in the past but on both occasions menstruation returned so she was not too concerned. Her periods started at the age of 12 years and were initially regular. She has no medical history of note and denies any medication. She is currently in her first year at university. She runs most days and reports a 'healthy' diet avoiding carbohydrate foods and meat. She is the oldest of three siblings and her parents separated when she was 12 years. She has minimal contact with her father and lives mainly with her mother who she says she gets on well with. She has had a boyfriend in the past but has veered away from any sexual relationships.

Examination

The woman is tall and thin with a BMI of 15.5 kg/m^2. There is evidence of fine downy hair growth on her arms. Heart rate is 86/min and blood pressure 100/65 mmHg. Abdominal examination reveals no scars or masses, and genital examination is not performed.

🔍 **INVESTIGATIONS**

		Normal Range
Follicle-stimulating hormone	1.0 IU/L	Day 2–5 1–11 IU/L
Luteinizing hormone	0.8 IU/L	Day 2–5 0.5–14.5 IU/L
Oestradiol	52 pmol/L	70–600 pmol/L
Prolactin	630 mu/L	90–520 mu/L
Testosterone	1.6 nmol/L	0.8–3.1 nmol/L

Transabdominal ultrasound report: The uterus is anteverted and measures 41 × 33 × 19 mm. The endometrium appears thin and regular measuring 2.3 mm.
The right ovary contains a few tiny follicles and the ovarian volume is 4.3 cm^3. The left ovary has no visible follicles and measures 3.8 cm^3. No dominant follicle or corpus luteum is visualized on either ovary.

? **QUESTIONS**

- What is the diagnosis?
- How would you further investigate and manage this woman?

DOI: 10.1201/9781003386933-20

ANSWER 19

The woman has evidence of hypogonadotrophic hypogonadism – she has low oestradiol levels associated with low gonadotrophin stimulation from the anterior pituitary. This may be due to various pituitary or hypothalamic causes, but in this case relates to anorexia nervosa and possibly excessive exercise. The raised prolactin is consistent with stress and does not need to be investigated further. At a BMI below 18 kg/m², menstruation tends to cease, returning once the BMI increases again (though often with several months' delay).

The ultrasound shows a small uterus, very thin inactive endometrium and immature ovaries with minimal follicular activity, all of which are typical findings in anorexia nervosa.

The previous episodes of amenorrhoea probably occurred when her dietary intake was very low and it may be that starting at university has increased her stress levels with the consequence of worsening her anorexia.

Further Investigation
- Full blood count, liver and renal function should all be monitored as these are affected in severe disease.
- A bone scan should be arranged to check for bone density – hypooestrogenism as a result of anorexia is likely to induce early-onset osteoporosis and fractures.
- Psychological assessment is also important to guide appropriate treatment.

Management
Encouraging the woman to eat a more normal diet and to avoid exercising is the ideal management, but anorexia is a chronic disease that is often refractory to treatment. Explanation that her periods will return if she increases her BMI may possibly encourage her to put on weight.

The combined oral contraceptive pill should be prescribed in the meantime, which will prevent osteoporosis and bring on periods, albeit pharmacologically induced.

Referral to a specialist eating disorders unit is vital in addressing the long-term problem for this woman. Commonly, eating disorders arise out of childhood difficulties and family or group therapy should be considered as part of a multidisciplinary treatment schedule.

If the investigations suggest renal or hepatic impairment then inpatient management is likely to be necessary.

 KEY POINTS

- Menstruation usually ceases when BMI is less than 18 kg/m².
- Amenorrhoeic anorexic women need oestrogen replacement to protect them from osteopaenia and subsequent osteoporosis.
- Anorexia is often refractory to treatment.

CASE 20: ABDOMINAL AND BACK PAIN

History

An 83-year-old woman complains of a dragging sensation in the lower abdomen and low back pain when standing or walking. It has been present for some years but she can now only stand for a short time before feeling uncomfortable. It is not noticeable at night. She has had four vaginal deliveries. She had her menopause at 52 years and took hormone replacement therapy for several years following this for vasomotor symptoms. She has not had any postmenopausal bleeding and has not had a smear for several years.

She is generally constipated and sometimes finds she can only defecate by placing her fingers into the vagina and compressing a 'bulge' she can feel. She has mild frequency and gets up twice most nights to pass urine. There is no dysuria or haematuria. Occasionally she does not get to the toilet in time and leaks a small amount of urine, but this does not worry her unduly.

Medically she is very well and does not take any medications regularly. She lives alone and does her own shopping and housework.

Examination

On examination she appears well. Blood pressure and heart rate are normal. She has a normal BMI. The abdomen is soft and non-tender. There is a loss of vulval anatomy consistent with atrophic changes. On examination in the supine position there is a mild prolapse. On standing, the cervix is felt at the level of the introitus. There is a large posterior wall prolapse and a minimal anterior wall prolapse.

? | **QUESTIONS**

- What is the diagnosis for her discomfort and pain?
- How could the prolapse be more thoroughly assessed?
- How would you manage this patient?

DOI: 10.1201/9781003386933-21

ANSWER 20

The diagnosis is of second-degree uterovaginal prolapse with rectocoele. Prolapse is traditionally categorized according to the level of descent of the cervix in relation to the introitus:

- *First degree*: Descent within the vagina
- *Second degree*: Descent to the introitus
- *Third degree*: Descent of the cervix outside the vagina
- *Procidentia*: Complete eversion of the vagina outside the introitus

A more thorough assessment using the Pelvic Organ Prolapse Quantification (POP-Q) System is now standard practice. It is a validated tool to quantify, describe and stage pelvic support. The hymen is used as the main reference point with measurements taken (and recorded on a grid) from six defined reference points plus three further measurements, with positive or negative numbers assigned according to whether the reference points are located above or below the hymen.

Common presenting symptoms are of 'something coming down', a 'lump' or a dragging sensation. Symptoms are always worse on standing or walking because of the effect of gravity. Prolapse is more common in women who are parous, have had long or traumatic deliveries, have a chronic cough or constipation. However it may occur in any woman, even if she is nulliparous, as it relates to collagen strength.

Management

Initial management involves treating the constipation with dietary manipulation and laxatives. This may relieve some of the symptoms and is also important to prevent recurrence if surgery is to be performed.

Pelvic floor exercises are helpful for mild prolapse and to preserve the integrity of repair postoperatively, though in this case they are unlikely to make any significant difference to the presenting symptoms. If surgery is not wanted then she can try a ring pessary (or shelf pessary if more uterine descent) to hold up the prolapse, which can work extremely well and only needs replacing every 6 months.

Although she is 83 this woman has no medical problems and should be offered definitive prolapse surgery which for her involves vaginal hysterectomy and posterior vaginal wall repair (colporrhaphy). As there is no abdominal incision involved, recovery is quick and she would expect to be in hospital for up to 3 days.

 KEY POINTS

- Prolapse incidence increases with age, parity, constipation and chronic cough.
- Conservative management with a ring pessary, or surgical prolapse repair may be appropriate.
- Relief of exacerbating factors is important to prevent symptoms worsening or to maintain the integrity of the repair.

CASE 21: POSTOPERATIVE CONFUSION

History

You are on call in the early evening and are asked to see a woman in the day surgery unit who is confused postoperatively. She is 42 years old and underwent transcervical resection of multiple submucosal fibroids in the early afternoon after presenting with menorrhagia. Four fibroids were resected and the estimated blood loss was 150 mL.

Examination

The woman knows her name but is disorientated, scoring only 5/10 on a mini-mental state examination. She seems slightly drowsy. She is of slight build and her preoperative weight was recorded as 57 kg. The heart rate is 100/min and the blood pressure is 105/70 mmHg. Oxygen saturation is 94 per cent on air. She is apyrexial. Chest examination reveals dullness at both bases with fine inspiratory crackles. The abdomen is not distended but there is generalized lower abdominal tenderness. No masses are palpable and there are no signs of peritonism. You can see that there is a small amount of blood on the sanitary pad, but the loss is not excessive. You are told that she passed urine an hour ago without difficulty.

The operation note is reviewed and you find that the procedure was essentially uncomplicated but was halted before all the fibroids could be fully resected because of the fluid imbalance. The fluid deficit is recorded as 1010 mL. However you review the actual fluid chart and it is as follows:

- *Fluid input (saline, via operating hysteroscope input channel)*: 1000 mL; 1000 mL; 1000 mL; 1000mL; 950 mL
- *Fluid output (via operating hysteroscope output channel)*: 1940 mL

INVESTIGATIONS

		Normal Range
Haemoglobin	104 g/L	117–157 g/L
Haematocrit	29%	36–58%
White cell count	7.1×10^9/L	$3.5–11 \times 10^9$/L
Platelets	302×10^9/L	$150–440 \times 10^9$/L
Sodium	129 mmol/L	135–145 mmol/L
Potassium	3.1 mmol/L	3.5–5 mmol/L
Urea	1.6 mmol/L	2.5–6.7 mmol/L
Creatinine	56 mmol/L	70–120 mmol/L

The chest X-ray is shown in Figure 21.1.

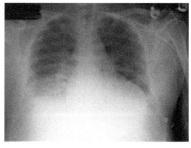

Figure 21.1 Chest X-ray.

? QUESTIONS

- What is the diagnosis and why has it occurred?
- How would you manage this patient?

DOI: 10.1201/9781003386933-22

ANSWER 21

The chest examination and X-ray suggest pulmonary oedema. Investigations show hyponatraemia and this is a recognized cause of a confusional state. There is also hypokalaemia which puts her at risk of dysrhythmia or cardiac arrest.

There has been an error in calculating the fluid deficit such that the deficit is in fact 3010 mL rather than 1010 mL. The hyponatraemia is therefore caused by fluid overload, a recognized complication of transcervical resection procedures. A fluid deficit of 2500 mL should be used as threshold to define fluid overload when using isotonic solutions such as saline in healthy women of reproductive age. In this particular case the impact of the excess fluid may be also exacerbated by her being of slighter build and therefore her own circulating volume will be lower.

Management

The mainstay of management is supportive with monitoring of electrolytes and fluid restriction. Potassium supplementation should be given and electrocardiogram (ECG) monitoring employed until the potassium is normal.

The woman should be transferred to a high-dependency bed and given oxygen. Arterial blood gas should be monitored, and if the pulmonary oedema worsens then diuretics will be needed.

The hyponatraemia usually corrects itself with time and fluid restriction, and the acute confusional state would be expected to resolve as the electrolytes normalize.

The fibroids were not completely resected and a repeat ultrasound or outpatient hysteroscopy may be considered after a few months to check whether further surgery is needed – sometimes degeneration may occur as a result of thermal damage or inflammation from the initial procedure. Alternatively, any fibroid remnants may be expelled spontaneously through the cervix and vagina.

 KEY POINTS

- Fluid overload and consequent hyponatraemia is a recognized complication of transcervical resection procedures.
- Accurate input/output monitoring is vital during this procedure.
- Treatment is supportive until electrolytes return to normal.

CASE 22: POSTMENOPAUSAL BLEEDING

History

A 58-year-old woman reports postmenopausal bleeding for 6 months. Initially she did not pay much attention to it but it now occurs most days. It is generally light but for a few days recently it was almost like a period. There is no associated pain. The woman has never married or been sexually active. She has no previous gynaecological history and has never had a smear test. She was diagnosed with type 2 diabetes 4 years ago for which she takes oral hypoglycaemics. However she is not very compliant with diet modification, and her blood glucose is not well controlled such that starting insulin is being considered.

Examination

The woman is obese with a BMI of 32 kg/m². Her blood pressure is 150/80 mmHg. The abdomen is non-tender, but due to her adiposity it is not possible to feel for abdominal masses.

External genital examination is unremarkable. Speculum and bimanual examination are not performed as she has never been sexually active.

Transvaginal ultrasound was not possible and a transabdominal ultrasound examination was therefore performed with a full bladder.

 INVESTIGATIONS

Transabdominal ultrasound report: The uterus is of normal size and anteverted. The endometrium could not be clearly visualized. Both ovaries appear normal. Ultrasound view was restricted by patient adiposity.

Examination under anaesthetic and hysteroscopy: The vagina and cervix appear normal. Hysteroscopy showed an irregular vascular mass arising from the uterine wall with contact bleeding. Curettage was performed and products sent for histological examination.

The findings at hysteroscopy are shown in Figure 22.1.

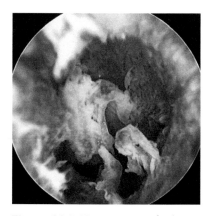

? QUESTIONS

- What is the likely diagnosis?
- If this is confirmed how would you manage this patient?

Figure 22.1 Hysteroscopy findings.

DOI: 10.1201/9781003386933-23

ANSWER 22

Postmenopausal bleeding should be considered to be due to endometrial carcinoma until proven otherwise. In many cases the diagnosis turns out to be benign. However in this case early suspicion is raised by the risk factors for endometrial carcinoma:

- Type 2 diabetes
- Obesity
- Nulliparity

There is also a long history of significant bleeding suggesting a more significant pathology. In women who can tolerate the examination, the diagnosis may be made by outpatient endometrial sampling. In this case, however, the inability to examine properly meant it was appropriate to investigate the uterine cavity and the rest of the lower genital tract under anaesthetic. The diagnosis of endometrial cancer was confirmed on histology report from the curettage specimen.

Management

Most (up to 90 per cent) of women with endometrial cancer have localized disease and are usually cured by hysterectomy and bilateral salpingoophorectomy. This is commonly carried out laparoscopically and increasingly with robotic assistance. Magnetic resonance imaging (MRI) scan prior to surgery should be carried out to check for depth of myometrial invasion and possible lymph node involvement, in which case lymph node biopsy or excision should be performed at the time of surgery. Formal staging is histological. Adjuvant radiotherapy is indicated if there is deep invasion of the myometrial muscle (50 per cent of the depth) or in grade 3 disease.

As with other gynaecology malignancies, these women should be looked after by a gynae-oncology multidisciplinary team comprising gynaecologists, oncologists, specialist nurses and in this case also the diabetic team.

! FIGO STAGING OF ENDOMETRIAL CARCINOMA			
Stage			**Prognosis (5-Year Survival Rate)**
I	IA	Tumour confined to the uterus, no or <50% myometrial invasion	85%
	IB	Tumour confined to the uterus, >50% myometrial invasion	
II		Cervical stromal invasion, but not beyond uterus	75%
III	IIIA	Tumour invades serosa or adnexa	45%
	IIIB	Vaginal and/or parametrial involvement	
	IIIC	Pelvic/para-aortic node involvement	
IV	IVA	Invasion into bladder and/or bowel mucosa	25%
	IVB	Distant metastases including abdominal metastases and/or inguinal lymph nodes	

🔑 | **KEY POINTS**

- Postmenopausal bleeding is due to endometrial cancer until proven otherwise.
- Women with risk factors or with prolonged or heavy bleeding are more likely to have pathology.
- Endometrial cancer is staged histologically.
- The majority of women present with stage I disease and have a good prognosis (85 per cent 5-year survival).

CASE 23: PELVIC PAIN

History

A 24-year-old woman presents with pelvic pain and painful sexual intercourse for 2 years. She is worried that she may have an ovarian cyst. The pain occurs at any time of the menstrual cycle but is worse during menstruation. It can also be worse when she passes urine or opens her bowels. There is no relation to exercise.

She has been with her current sexual partner for 6 months and the pain occurs nearly every time she has intercourse unless penetration is very gentle. She has never been diagnosed with any sexually transmitted infections. She was pregnant once at the age of 19 years but this ended in a spontaneous complete miscarriage.

She opens her bowels regularly and denies any bloating, constipation, diarrhoea or mucus in the stool. She had an episode of what she described as cystitis a few years ago which responded to antibiotics.

There is no other medical history of note and she takes no regular medications.

Examination

The abdomen is not distended and there is no organomegaly. No masses are palpable but there is suprapubic tenderness. Speculum examination shows a normal smooth grey/white coloured discharge and swabs are taken. The uterus is anteverted but has limited mobility and is tender on movement. There are no adnexal masses but the adnexae are tender.

 INVESTIGATIONS

Urinalysis: Protein negative; blood negative; leucocytes negative; nitrites negative
Endocervical chlamydia swab: Negative
High vaginal swab: Negative
Transvaginal ultrasound report: The uterus is normal sized and axial. The endometrium measures 12 mm. Both ovaries are of normal morphology but appear adherent to the posterior uterus and show limited mobility. There is no free fluid in the pouch of Douglas

Laparoscopy findings are shown in Figures 23.1 and 23.2.

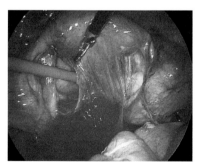

Figure 23.1 Laparoscopy image of the pelvis.

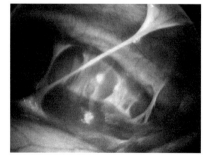

Figure 23.2 Laparoscopy image of the right upper abdomen.

? **QUESTIONS**

- What is the diagnosis?
- How would you manage this patient?
- What are the long-term implications of this disease?

DOI: 10.1201/9781003386933-24

ANSWER 23

The laparoscopy image in Figure 23.1 shows pelvic adhesions suggestive of previous infection. The 'violin-string' perihepatic adhesions in Figure 23.2 are classical of Fitz–Hugh–Curtis syndrome, generally seen with previous chlamydial infection though also described with gonorrhoea. These findings can develop in the absence of a clinically recognized infective episode.

The woman therefore has chronic pain from pelvic inflammatory disease. Negative swabs would suggest that she may no longer be infected with chlamydia.

Management

The pain may be helped with laparoscopic adhesiolysis. The perihepatic adhesions should be ignored as they are not causing symptoms. Otherwise pain-management options are analgesics or if chronic symptoms persist then a multidisciplinary pain management team assessment including psychology and physiotherapy input.

Even though there is no evidence of current active infection, the tests have limited sensitivity so it is worthwhile treating the woman and her partner with a course of antibiotics for pelvic inflammatory disease.

❗ LONG-TERM COMPLICATIONS OF PELVIC INFLAMMATORY DISEASE

- Chronic pain.
- Infertility: Tubal infertility is likely in this woman, and if she fails to conceive spontaneously then hysterosalpingogram or hysterosalpingo-constrast sonography (HyCoSy) should be performed with referral for assisted conception if tubal obstruction is confirmed.
- Ectopic pregnancy: Spontaneous and *in vitro* fertilization pregnancies are at increased risk of implanting in the damaged tubes, and an early transvaginal scan should be advised if she becomes pregnant.
- The woman should also be advised that despite the likely subfertility, spontaneous pregnancy may still occur so she should use effective contraception if she does not want to conceive.

🔑 KEY POINTS

- Fitz–Hugh–Curtis syndrome is the presence of perihepatic adhesions in association with previous chlamydial or gonococcal infection.
- Treatment of both partners is appropriate.
- Chronic pain, ectopic pregnancy and tubal infertility are long-term consequences of pelvic inflammatory disease.

CASE 24: PRIMARY AMENORRHOEA

History

A 14-year-old girl is seen by her general practitioner because her mother is worried that her periods have not started. Her older sister started at 13 years and her younger sister has just started her periods at 12 years, and she is now embarrassed at school as her friends are always discussing their periods and she has not told them that she has not had one.

Her mother is also concerned because she has not developed pubic and axillary hair or breast enlargement.

She was born at 38 weeks by spontaneous vaginal delivery and has never had any particular medical problems. She reached all her developmental milestones as a child, although has not started a teenage growth spurt and is now the second shortest girl in her class.

She eats normally with her family and denies any eating disorder. She takes part in school sport but does not exercise to excess.

She is sociable with her friends but has never had a boyfriend.

Her school academic performance is about average, although she does not do as well as her siblings who are all in the top streams of their years.

Examination

On examination she is 120 cm and weighs 59 kg. She has no abnormal facial features but has a wide carrying angle (cubitus valgus) and a wide neck. There is no apparent breast development and the nipples appear widely spaced. No axillary hair growth is apparent.

Abdominal examination is unremarkable. The external genitalia are normal though no pubic hair is visible. Internal examination is not performed.

🔍 INVESTIGATIONS

		Normal Range
Follicle-stimulating hormone	24 IU/L	1–11 IU/L
Luteinizing hormone	20 IU/L	0.5–14.5 IU/L
Oestradiol	84 pmol/L	70–510 pmol/L
Prolactin	239 mu/L	90–520 mu/L
Karyotype: 45 XO		
Free thyroxine	17 pmol/L	11–23 pmol/L

Transabdominal ultrasound report: The uterus appears small and anteverted. The endometrium appears smooth and thin, measuring 2.4 mm. Both ovaries are visualized and appear to be of small volume. No follicles are seen.

? QUESTIONS

- What is the most likely diagnosis and how might this be confirmed?
- What are the principles of management for this girl?

DOI: 10.1201/9781003386933-25

ANSWER 24

The clinical features are typical of those of monosomy X (Turner's syndrome). This genetic condition is associated with the absence of one X chromosome (45 XO karyotype), occurring in approximately 1 in 2500 live female births. It is confirmed on chromosomal analysis.

In rare cases it may occur as a mosaic form (XX/XO), in which case the features are milder and the woman may start menstruating but then experience premature ovarian insufficiency and secondary amenorrhoea. Occasionally these women are able to conceive. These pregnancies need to be treated as high risk due to the possibility of aortic aneurysm.

> **! COMMON CLINICAL FEATURES OF TURNER'S SYNDROME**
>
> • Webbed neck
> • Broad chest with widely spaced nipples ('shield chest')
> • Wide carrying angle (cubitus valgus)
> • Short stature (maximum 150 cm without treatment)
> • Short fourth metacarpal
> • Low-set ears
> • Low hairline
> • Hypoplastic nails
> • Hypertension
> • Congenital heart disease (e.g. coarctation of the aorta)

Management

Management of Turner's syndrome should be carried out in a specialist referral centre.

- *Psychological*: The implications of Turner's syndrome diagnosis are devastating for the child and for the family. The absence of periods may be stigmatizing and the long-term lack of fertility is a very serious concept that may be difficult for a young girl to comprehend.
- *Medical*: The short stature should be treated to enable the girl to reach her full height potential. Human growth hormone is given to achieve this under the supervision of an endocrinologist.
  - Oestrogen therapy initially with ethinyl estradiol enables secondary sexual characteristics of breast development and pubic and axillary hair to develop. Cyclical progestogens are added later to induce a withdrawal bleed ('period') for social reasons and to protect the endometrium from hyperplasia or malignancy in the long term. Some form of oestrogen therapy then needs to be continued until the time of natural menopause (ideally 50 years) to prevent early-onset osteoporosis.
- *Fertility*: Fertility options are available with ovum donation and hormonal support.

> **🔑 KEY POINTS**
>
> • Turner's syndrome is a cause of primary amenorrhoea.
> • Most girls will be diagnosed in early childhood because of small stature or other physical features, but some will only be diagnosed when menarche fails to occur.
> • Treatment, usually hormonal, to protect bone density is essential.

CASE 25: PERMANENT CONTRACEPTION

History

A couple attends the antenatal clinic requesting sterilization. They have three children, aged 10, 7 and 5, all born by caesarean section. The oldest son has Asperger's syndrome. Until now they have been using the contraceptive pill but as the woman is slightly overweight (BMI 29 kg/m²) and has a family history of cardiovascular disease, her GP has advised her to seek an alternative. She tried the levonorgestrel-releasing intrauterine system but had it removed after 6 months due to irregular bleeding.

She is aged 38 and is otherwise healthy. She does not smoke and takes no other medication.

Her husband is supportive and initially planned a vasectomy but after initial consultation decided that he could not go through with it due to his fear of the procedure.

They have read widely on the Internet and decided that laparoscopic sterilization is the most suitable method for them in view of its reliability and permanence.

Examination

Blood pressure is 150/85 mmHg. On abdominal inspection the caesarean section scars are noted as well as an appendectomy scar.

The abdomen is soft and non-tender with no palpable masses. Speculum examination is unremarkable and on bimanual examination the uterus is normal sized, mobile and anteverted.

?	QUESTIONS
	• How would you establish whether sterilization really is an appropriate choice for this couple?
	• If you agree with her request for laparoscopic sterilization in principle, how would you counsel regarding the procedure before agreeing to proceed?
	• Are there any other suitable contraceptive options that this woman should consider apart from laparoscopic sterilization?

DOI: 10.1201/9781003386933-26

ANSWER 25

Appropriateness of Sterilization

The fact that this couple's youngest child is 5 years old would suggest that they have had time to consider having further children and have definitively decided against this. It may be that the eldest child with Asperger's means that they are particularly keen to avoid pregnancy due to their involvement with his care. However in counselling couples regarding sterilization, it is important to encourage them to consider whether there are any circumstances under which their decision might change, e.g. the death of an existing child (or children) or the breakup of their relationship and wanting to have a child with a new partner.

Assuming that these have been considered and other non-permanent contraceptive options offered, or as in this case of the levonorgestrel-releasing intrauterine system having been tried, then sterilization is a reasonable and effective choice.

Counselling before Laparoscopic Sterilization

In addition to an explanation of the laparoscopic sterilization procedure, the following points should be discussed and documented before consent for sterilization is obtained:

- Sterilization should be considered a permanent procedure. Reversal of tubal sterilization has low success rates (maximum 60 per cent) and neither this nor IVF would be eligible for NHS funding.
- Up to 10 per cent of women regret their decision for sterilization.
- The failure rate of laparoscopic sterilization is quoted as 2 in 100 women who have been sterilized for one year – this is significantly higher than male sterilization (1 in 2000 failure rate).
- If a pregnancy does occur after sterilization then there is an increased risk of this being an ectopic pregnancy. Early ultrasound scan is therefore recommended in such circumstances.
- Laparoscopy carries associated risks of bleeding, infection, injury to bowel or bladder or blood vessels (3 in 1000 risk of significant harm), thrombosis and anaesthetic complications. These risks may be increased in this case due to the woman's previous surgery, blood pressure and BMI.
- There is a small chance that sterilization procedure will be impossible due to technical difficulty which would need conversion to an open procedure. In this case as she has previously had three caesarean sections there is a possibility that the tubes will not be accessible at all due to adhesions and the sterilization abandoned.

CASE 26: LABILE MOOD AND ABDOMINAL PAIN

History

A 37-year-old mother presents to her general practitioner with cyclical labile mood swings. She says that she has always suffered with premenstrual syndrome (PMS) and that it is in the family as her mother 'had to have a hysterectomy' for the same problem. She reports her periods as always having been painful and that she has always been irritable leading up to a period. However now she feels that she is not herself for at least 2 weeks before her period and that the pain has worsened. She also notices headaches, swelling and breast tenderness.

Her periods are generally regular with bleeding for up to 6 days every 27–31 days. She has had three children all by normal vaginal delivery and the youngest is now 5 years old. She has no other medical history of note.

She has been married for 14 years and she says she often feels aggressive towards her husband or alternatively is tearful and low. Prior to having children she worked in a bank and is not sure whether to return as she feels she might be unable to cope.

Examination

No abnormality is found on abdominal or neurological examination.

? | **QUESTIONS**

- What is the differential diagnosis?
- How would you further determine the cause of the symptoms and manage this patient?

DOI: 10.1201/9781003386933-27

ANSWER 26

The woman clearly feels that this is a gynaecological problem and that she has PMS. The diagnosis should be confirmed with evidence of symptoms occurring in the luteal phase and resolving within a day or two of menstruation starting. The differential diagnosis is depression which can manifest in a similar way to PMS.

A symptom diary is needed for recording symptoms for each day, over 2 cycles. The woman should annotate a chart with the severity of each symptom and when menstruation occurs. PMS should start after midcycle, symptoms should resolve with the period and there should be a number of symptom-free days each month. If there is doubt about diagnosis GnRH analogues can be used to aid diagnosis. Where symptoms are very severe the term premenstrual dysphoric disorder (PMDD) is used.

An example of a symptom diary is shown in Figure 26.1.

Management

If confirmed then the diagnosis should be discussed with the woman, offering appropriate understanding and support but explaining that management is variable in terms of success for each woman and that 'one size does not fit all'. Exercise, cognitive behavioural therapy and vitamin B6 have been shown to have benefit in PMS and should be offered as a first line.

Interruption of ovulation with the oral contraceptive pill is often successful in women under the age of 35 years. Evidence now suggests that this can be taken continuously rather than cyclically in a so-called 'back to back' approach.

Selective serotonin reuptake inhibitors taken continuously or only in the luteal phase have a good success rate in randomized trials, and the woman should be advised that they have a specific effect with PMS rather than just a general antidepressant effect. There is limited evidence for the role of continuous oestrogens or progestogens for the management of PMS.

In cases resistant to other treatments, a therapeutic trial of gonadotrophin-releasing hormone analogues to induce a pseudomenopause can be considered, though the associated hypoestrogenic side effects may themselves need treating with added-back oestrogen. If this is used as a long-term solution the woman would need a bone scan yearly.

Hysterectomy would not be helpful unless the ovaries were also removed, and this would involve risk of significant morbidity with the need for hormone replacement therapy afterwards which may have its own side effects or complications, although in very severe and refractory cases this may be necessary.

 KEY POINTS

- Premenstrual syndrome is diagnosed with a symptom diary.
- Severe premenstrual syndrome is known as premenstrual dysphoric disorder (PMDD).
- No single treatment is effective for all women.
- Selective serotonin reuptake inhibitors are effective in many women with premenstrual syndrome.

Symptom diary

May

Symptom	1	2	3	4	5	6	7	8	9	10	11	12	13	14	15	16	17	18	19	20	21	22	23	24	25	26	27	28	29	30	31
Breast tenderness	xxx	xxx	xx	xx	xx	x																	x	x	x	xx	xx	xxx	xxx	xxx	xx
Low mood	xxxx	xxxx	x	xxxx	xxx	xxx	x																		x	xx	x	x	x	xx	xxx
Feeling aggressive	xxxx	xx	xx	xxxx	xx																							x		x	x
Bloated	x	x	xx	xx	x	x	x															xx	xx	xx	xxx	xxx	x	x	xx	x	xx
Menstruation						x	x	x	x	x	x	x																			

June

Symptom	1	2	3	4	5	6	7	8	9	10	11	12	13	14	15	16	17	18	19	20	21	22	23	24	25	26	27	28	29	30
Breast tenderness	x	xx																x	x	xx	xx	xxx	x	x	xx	xxx	xxx	xxx	xxx	x
Low mood	xxx		x								x													x	xx	xxx	xxx	xxx	xxx	xxx
Feeling aggressive	x																			x		x	x			x	x	xxx	xx	xx
Bloated	xx	xx	x																											
Menstruation		x	x	x	x	x	x	x																						x

July

Symptom	1	2	3	4	5	6	7	8	9	10	11	12	13	14	15	16	17	18	19	20	21	22	23	24	25	26	27	28	29	30	31
Breast tenderness																x	xx	xx	x	xx	xx	x	xxx	x	x						
Low mood	x						x									xxx	xxx	xxx	xxx	xxx	xxx	xxxx	xxxx	xx	xx	xx	xx				
Feeling aggressive	x																			x	x	xx	x	x							
Bloated	x	x														x	xx	xx	xxx	xxx	x	x	x	xxx	xxx	xx	xx	x	x	x	
Menstruation	x	x	x	xx																								x	x	x	x

Figure 26.1 Premenstrual syndrome symptom diary.

CASE 27: CERVICAL CANCER

History

A 28-year-old woman was referred to the colposcopy clinic because of intermenstrual and post-coital bleeding. On examination a macroscopically visible lesion was present and on colposcopy features of malignancy were seen. Subsequent biopsy showed invasive squamous carcinoma of the cervix.

The woman was informed of the diagnosis and as a result went on to undergo an examination under anaesthetic, cystoscopy and proctoscopy for staging. The mass was found to be 3 cm in size and there was no palpable extension into the uterus, vagina or parametrial tissues. The cystoscopy and proctoscopy were both normal.

 INVESTIGATIONS

		Normal Range
Haemoglobin	120 g/L	117–157 g/L
White cell count	8 × 10⁹/L	3.5–11 × 10⁹/L
Platelets	344 × 10⁹/L	150–440 × 10⁹/L
Sodium	138 mmol/L	135–145 mmol/L
Potassium	3.5 mmol/L	3.5–5 mmol/L
Urea	3.6 mmol/L	2.5–6.7 mmol/L
Creatinine	76 mmol/L	70–120 mmol/L

Chest X-ray report: Normal heart and lung fields. No abnormalities detected.
Renal tract ultrasound report: Normal-sized kidneys. Both ureters are of normal calibre with no evidence of obstruction.

She has had one child but had been hoping to have at least one more and is devastated by the diagnosis.

? **QUESTION**

• What are the possible treatment options and their potential complications?

DOI: 10.1201/9781003386933-28

ANSWER 27

Cervical cancer may be treated surgically or by radiotherapy. Staging is performed clinically at examination under anaesthetic as described.

! CERVICAL CANCER STAGING			
Staging			*Prognosis (5-Year Survival)*
I Confined to cervix	IA1	Microscopic lesion. Invasion <3 mm depth and lateral spread <7 mm	95%
	IA2	Microscopic lesion. Invasion >3 mm and <5 mm with lateral spread <7 mm	
	IB1	Clinically visible lesion <4 cm in greatest dimension	80%
	IB2	Clinically visible lesion >4 cm in greatest dimension	
II Invades beyond uterus but not to pelvic wall or lower 1/3 of vagina	IIA1	Involves upper 2/3 of vagina, without parametrial invasion, <4 cm in greatest dimension	60%
	IIA2	Involves upper 2/3 of vagina, without parametrial invasion, >4 cm in greatest dimension	
	IIB	With parametrial involvement	
III Extends to pelvic wall and/or involves lower 1/3 of vagina and/or causes hydronephrosis or non-functioning kidney	IIIA	Involves lower 1/3 of vagina with no extension to the pelvic wall	35%
	IIIB	Extension to pelvic wall and/or hydronephrosis or non-functioning kidney	
IV Extension beyond true pelvis or involves mucosa of bladder or rectum	IVA	Spread of the growth to adjacent organs	15%
	IVB	Spread to distant organs	

Radical Hysterectomy

Up to stage IB women may be treated with radical hysterectomy (also known as Wertheim's hysterectomy). This involves removal of the uterus, cervix, pelvic lymph nodes and parametrial tissue as well as the upper third of the vagina. Complications involve bleeding and infection. Ureteric damage may occur and blood vessel injury is not uncommon. Postoperative complications include infections of the chest, wound or urinary tract as well as venous thromboembolism and later-onset lymphoedema from interruption of lymphatic drainage from the lower limbs.

The advantage of this treatment is that it preserves ovarian function, important for wellbeing and prevention of osteoporosis. It also avoids the complications of radiotherapy outlined below.

Trachelectomy

This involves removal of the cervix, lymph nodes and parametrial tissue with conservation of the ovaries and uterine body with insertion of a suture (cerclage) at the base of the uterus. It is used selectively for women with early stage disease who wish to preserve their fertility.

Radiotherapy

Disease beyond stage IB, and postmenopausal women should be treated with radiotherapy which is effective but is associated with long-term effects of bowel stenosis, cystitis and vaginal stenosis. It also generally renders women menopausal due to radiation to the ovaries.

 KEY POINTS

- Cervical carcinoma should be considered in any woman with intermenstrual or post-coital bleeding.
- Disease staging is clinical, under anaesthetic.
- Cervical carcinoma may be treated surgically or by radiotherapy, depending on the stage of disease.

CASE 28: URINARY INCONTINENCE

History

A 49-year-old woman presents with leaking of urine. This started after the birth of her third child 10 years ago and has gradually worsened. She has not felt comfortable talking to her general practitioner about it until now. The leakage occurs on coughing and laughing. However she has recently started to play badminton to lose weight and the symptoms are much worse, but she has discovered that the symptoms are much better if she wears a tampon while playing. There is no dysuria, nocturia, frequency or urgency. She is mildly constipated.

All her children were born by induction of labour post-term. They weighed 3.6 kg, 3.8 kg and 4.1 kg, respectively, and she needed a forceps delivery for the first child after failure to progress in the second stage of labour. She has a regular menstrual cycle and has had a laparoscopic sterilization. There is no other relevant medical history and she takes no medications. She smokes 15 cigarettes per day and does not drink alcohol.

Examination

BMI is 29 kg/m^2. There are no significant findings on abdominal or vaginal examination.

 INVESTIGATIONS

Urinalysis: Protein negative; blood negative; leucocytes negative; nitrites negative.
Urodynamics report: The first urge to void was felt at 300 mL. The maximum bladder capacity was 450 mL. Involuntary loss of urine was noted with coughing during bladder filling, in the absence of detrusor activity.

? QUESTIONS

- What is the diagnosis?
- How would you advise and manage this woman?

DOI: 10.1201/9781003386933-29

ANSWER 28

This woman is suffering from stress incontinence. Stress incontinence can be diagnosed from the history – involuntary loss of urine when the intra-abdominal pressure increases (such as with exercise or coughing). Urodynamic stress incontinence (formerly referred to as genuine stress incontinence) is the involuntary loss of urine when the intravesical pressure exceeds the maximum urethral pressure in the absence of a detrusor contraction and can only be diagnosed after urodynamic testing.

Management

Conservative Management

- *Lifestyle*: The woman should be advised to control factors that exacerbate symptoms:
  - Reduce weight.
  - Stop smoking to relieve chronic cough symptoms.
  - Alter diet and consider laxatives to avoid constipation.
- *Pelvic floor exercises*: Properly taught pelvic floor muscle training is a very effective treatment and can cause improvement in symptoms or cure in up to 85 per cent of women.

Surgical Management

Colposuspension

This open or laparoscopic procedure involves sutures to lift the vagina which then supports the urethra, reducing leakage.

Bulking Injections

Periurethral injection of bulking agents (such as collagen) may be used in refractory cases or for women unfit for surgery. These agents augment the urethral wall and increase resistance to urinary leakage.

Tension-Free Vaginal Tape or Transobturator Tape

These minimally invasive techniques (known as mid-urethral sling procedures) involve insertion of a tape to support the urethra and bladder when the intra-abdominal pressure increases (such as during coughing). The TOT (which uses the obturator route) is associated with a slightly lower rate of perforation of the bladder or vagina and of voiding difficulty when compared to the TVT (which uses the retropubic route) but may result in a higher chance of groin pain or erosion of the tape into the vagina. These procedures are carried out infrequently now and only at specialist centres due to complications that have arisen in some women who have undergone such mesh procedures in the past.

Medical Management

Duloxetine is a serotonin-norepinephrine reuptake inhibitor (SNRI) which reduces the frequency of episodes of stress incontinence in women declining or otherwise unsuitable for surgical management.

A bladder diary should be recorded before and after any intervention to aid assessment of effectiveness.

 KEY POINTS

- Stress incontinence is a clinical diagnosis.
- First-line treatment is avoidance of exacerbating factors and pelvic muscle exercises.
- Urodynamic stress incontinence should be confirmed prior to surgery.

CASE 29: PELVIC PAIN

History

A 21-year-old student presents with left iliac fossa and lower abdominal pain. The pain is present intermittently with no pattern except that it is generally worse on exercise and so she has stopped running to keep fit. The pain started about 6 months before and has gradually become more frequent and severe. It is no worse with her periods and she is not currently sexually active so cannot report any dyspareunia. Her periods are regular and not particularly heavy or painful. She has no previous gynaecological problems. She has had one sexual partner who she was with for 4 years. She has not had any sexually transmitted infections.

Medically she is fit and well, and has only been admitted to hospital for wisdom teeth removal and for tonsillectomy as a child. She takes no medications.

Examination

The woman is slim and the abdomen is soft with a palpable mass in the left iliac fossa. This is firm and feels mobile. It is moderately tender.

Speculum examination is normal. Bimanual examination confirms an 8 cm mass in the left adnexa. The uterus is palpable separately and is mobile and anteverted. The right adnexa is normal.

 INVESTIGATIONS

An abdominal X-ray is shown in Figure 29.1.

Transvaginal ultrasound scan findings are shown in Figure 29.2.

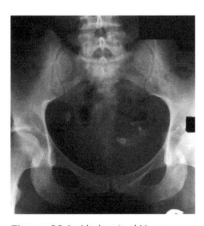

Figure 29.1 Abdominal X-ray.

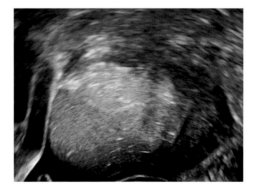

Figure 29.2 Transvaginal ultrasound image showing a transverse view through the left adnexa.

? **QUESTIONS**

- What is the diagnosis?
- How would you manage this woman?

DOI: 10.1201/9781003386933-30

ANSWER 29

The woman has a palpable left adnexal mass, which is shown on ultrasound to be a complex ovarian cyst. The appearance is of mixed echogenicity with 'acoustic shadowing' and this appearance is typical for a dermoid cyst (also known as a benign teratoma). Some normal ovarian tissue containing follicles can be seen adjacent to the cyst. The X-ray shows the presence of teeth in the left iliac fossa region.

These cysts are common and very often asymptomatic, picked up as an incidental finding. Typically sebaceous fluid is present, often in association with strands of hair or sometimes teeth. If active thyroid tissue develops the woman may present with features of hyperthyroidism and the cyst is referred to as a struma ovarii.

The management is surgical with ovarian cystectomy, due to the size of the cyst and the symptoms. Ideally this can be performed laparoscopically. In asymptomatic smaller cysts there is a possibility of expectant management ('watch and wait'). However, the risks of leaving the cyst are:

- Malignancy occurs in possibly up to 2 per cent of dermoid cysts.
- Ovarian torsion is thought to be relatively common in women with dermoid cysts, and if this occurs it is a medical emergency, which may involve oophorectomy.

The woman should be advised that the cysts are common and there is very little chance that it is malignant or that removing it will affect her fertility. However, recurrence may occur in either ovary and she should seek further consultation if she develops recurrent pain.

 KEY POINTS

- Dermoid cysts (mature cystic teratoma) are a common cause of ovarian cysts in young women.
- They commonly display a classic appearance on X-ray or ultrasound scan.
- Surgery is usually recommended because of a small risk of torsion or malignant transformation.

CASE 30: EARLY MENARCHE

History

An 8-year-old girl is referred by the general practitioner because her periods have started. She was born at term by spontaneous vaginal delivery after an uneventful pregnancy. She has had the normal childhood illnesses but there is no significant serious medical history of note. She takes no medication. Her physical development has been unremarkable until a year ago when she changed from being average height to the second tallest in her class.

Educationally she is achieving at a similar level to her peers. She has many friends and no behavioural problems. She is the first of three children and her mother reports her own period starting at 11 years.

Examination

General examination is normal. The girl has significant breast bud development and some fine pubic hair. Further genital examination is not performed.

> **? QUESTIONS**
> - What is the diagnosis and what are the problems associated with it?
> - How would you investigate and manage this girl?

DOI: 10.1201/9781003386933-31

ANSWER 30

The average age of menarche is 13 years, and the start of periods before the age of 9 years, as in this case, is classified as precocious puberty.

In normal puberty, girls tend to start breast bud development from 9–13 years, start pubic hair growth from 10–14 years and menarche starts at 11–15 years. An increased rate of growth starts at 11–12 years and growth finishes at around 15 years. When these changes occur early but in the normal sequence, the precocious puberty is usually of no significant consequence and termed constitutional early development. This is often familial. However, if it occurs very early or in an abnormal sequence, a pathological cause is more likely.

! CAUSES OF PRECOCIOUS PUBERTY

- Constitutional (>90 per cent)
- Hypothyroidism
- CNS lesions (hydrocephaly, neurofibromatosis)
- Ovarian tumour
- Adrenal tumour
- Exogenous oestrogens

Problems of Precocious Puberty

- *Growth*: Although the growth spurt starts early in precocious puberty, growth also stops prematurely (premature epiphyseal closure) and therefore girls with precocious puberty are at risk of having a reduced final stature if untreated.
- *Embarrassment*: Early secondary sexual characteristics and the onset of periods can be very difficult for a girl to deal with at a young age.
- *Social interaction*: Difficulties can occur when people who do not know the child's chronological age assume a level of intellectual and emotional maturity according to the child's physical maturity (apparent age).

Investigation

Gonadotrophins, prolactin and thyroid hormones should be checked to confirm that they correlate with normal pubertal levels. Computerized tomography (CT) or magnetic resonance imaging (MRI) may be necessary for visualization of the pituitary stalk. Abdominopelvic ultrasound will rule out an ovarian or adrenal tumour. Bone scan will determine biological bone age to ascertain whether pituitary suppression is indicated.

Management

As the changes in this girl seem to be in a normal sequence and she is within 2 years of the normal age of menarche she can be managed expectantly. However if the changes had started at a younger age, pituitary suppression should be started with gonadotrophin-releasing hormone analogues, to delay the growth spurt and thus maintain full final height.

🔑 KEY POINTS

- Over 90 per cent of girls with precocious puberty have constitutional (idiopathic) precocious puberty with no pathological cause, but an abnormal sequence of pubertal development or very early puberty should trigger further investigation.
- The major problems of precocious puberty are short final stature and social embarrassment.

CASE 31: EXCESSIVE HAIR GROWTH

History

A 19-year-old woman was referred by her general practitioner (GP) with increased body hair growth.

She first noticed the problem when she was about 16 years old and it has progressively worsened such that she now feels very self-conscious and will never wear a bikini or go swimming. It also affects her forming relationships. The hair growth is noticed mainly on her arms, thighs and abdomen. Hair has developed on the upper lip more recently. She has tried shaving but this seems to make the problem worse. She feels depilation creams are ineffective. Waxing is helpful but very expensive and she has bleached her upper-lip hair. Her GP has not prescribed any medication in the past.

There is no significant previous medical history of note. Her periods started at the age of 13 years and she bleeds every 30–35 days. The periods are not painful or heavy and there is no intermenstrual bleeding or discharge. She has never been sexually active.

Examination

On examination she has an increased BMI of 29 kg/m². The blood pressure is 118/70 mmHg. There is excessive hair growth on the lower arms, legs and thighs and in the midline of the abdomen below the umbilicus. There is a small amount of growth on the upper lip too. The abdomen is soft and no masses are palpable. Pelvic examination is not indicated as she has not been sexually active.

INVESTIGATIONS

		Normal Range
Follicle-stimulating hormone (FSH)	7 IU/L	Day 2–5 1–11 IU/L
Luteinizing hormone (LH)	12 IU/L	Day 2–5 0.5–14.5 IU/L
Prolactin	780 mu/L	90–520 mu/L
Testosterone	3.2 nmol/L	0.8–3.1 nmol/L
Thyroid-stimulating hormone	4.9 mu/L	0.5–5.7 mu/L
Free thyroxine	14.7 pmol/L	10–40 pmol/L

QUESTIONS

- What is the likely diagnosis?
- How would you further investigate and manage this woman?

DOI: 10.1201/9781003386933-32

ANSWER 31

The likely diagnosis is of polycystic ovarian syndrome (PCOS). This is supported by the clinical features of hirsutism, acne, increased BMI and slight menstrual irregularity. The biochemical results show the typical moderately raised androgen and raised LH:FSH ratio.

If the testosterone level was higher, androgen-secreting tumours should be considered (andro-gen-secreting ovarian, pituitary or adrenal tumours).

Other causes of hyperandrogenism include iatrogenic (glucocorticoids, danazol, testosterone), idiopathic or familial.

Further Investigation

A transabdominal ultrasound scan should be arranged to confirm the ultrasound features of polycystic ovaries, although this is not in fact an essential feature for the diagnosis of the syndrome.

Treatment

Various treatments are used for hirsutism once serious causes of hyperandrogenism have been excluded. One of the commonest is to commence the cyproterone acetate-containing combined oral contraceptive pill (co-cyprindiol). Cyproterone acetate is an antiandrogen with progesto-genic activity. It takes several months for an improvement to be seen in the hair growth and she would continue to need to use the cosmetic treatments in the meantime. She should be advised that the venous thrombosis risk with co-cyprindiol is slightly higher than with some other com-bined contraceptive pills and advised of the typical symptoms (painful swollen leg, chest pain or shortness of breath).

If this is ineffective then cyproterone acetate at a higher dose can be used either alone or in addi-tion to co-cyprindiol.

General advice should include weight loss, as this counteracts the metabolic imbalance associ-ated with PCOS and is favourable in the long term in terms of the known cardiovascular risks associated with hyperandrogenism. Laser hair removal is currently the most helpful treatment for cosmetic benefit with hirsutism, but may need to be repeated.

 KEY POINTS

- Most women with hirsutism have PCOS or a familial tendency.
- Androgen-secreting tumours should be excluded in women with testosterone level above 5 nmol/L.
- Hirsutism has significant psychosocial consequences.

Section 2
EMERGENCY GYNAECOLOGY

CASE 32: PAIN AND THE INTRAUTERINE SYSTEM

History

A 30-year-old woman had a levonorgestrel-releasing intrauterine system (IUS) inserted by her general practitioner 3 weeks ago. Ten days ago she presented to the emergency department with abdominal pain, and on examination the threads were not visible and ultrasound scan suggested the IUS was misplaced in the right uterine cornu. An appointment was made for hysteroscopic resection but she has presented again in the interim with further pain.

Examination

The abdomen is not distended and is soft. There is generalized lower abdominal tenderness. The threads cannot be visualized on speculum examination.

 INVESTIGATIONS

Transvaginal ultrasound report: The uterus is anteverted and of normal size. The endometrium is regular and measures 11 mm. An IUS is not visible. Both ovaries appear normal in size and morphology.

Abdominal X-ray is shown in Figure 32.1.

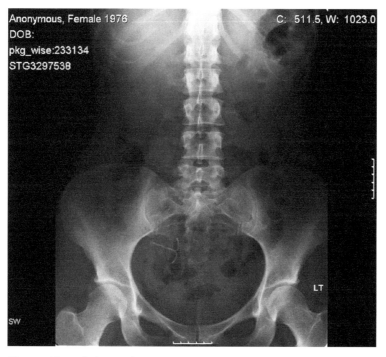

Figure 32.1 Abdominal X-ray.

? **QUESTIONS**

- How would you explain the symptoms and investigation findings?
- How would you further investigate and manage this patient?

DOI: 10.1201/9781003386933-34

ANSWER 32

The plain X-ray shows the IUS in the pelvis but it is lying at a transverse angle in the right pelvis. In this high and lateral location and at this orientation it is highly unlikely that the device is within the uterus, especially as the ultrasound report suggests a normal sized uterus. The current ultrasound result confirms that the uterus is empty. However the previous report suggested the device was at the uterine cornu. It can be concluded therefore that the device was inserted into the uterus but it has subsequently migrated through the myometrium into the peritoneal cavity. We have no evidence to determine whether or not it was originally placed in the correct position at the fundus.

> **!   COMPLICATIONS OF INTRAUTERINE CONTRACEPTIVE DEVICE (IUCD)/ INTRAUTERINE DEVICE INSERTION**
>
> - Uterine perforation
> - Device migration through to peritoneal cavity
> - Pelvic inflammatory disease
> - Expulsion of device (commonly with the next period)

Investigation

The only important investigation is a pregnancy test, as the woman is potentially pregnant since the IUS may not have been effective if it was never in the correct location.

Management

The IUS needs to be retrieved. While it was in the uterus this could have been performed with outpatient hysteroscopic retrieval. However, now a laparoscopy is indicated.

In this case the laparoscopy revealed blood-stained free fluid in the pouch of Douglas, with scarring on the right fundal area of the uterus. The IUS was found covered with omentum in the right lower abdomen. It was easily removed laparoscopically.

As the woman had wanted the IUS for contraception as well as treatment of her menorrhagia, and as the uterus appeared to have healed, a new IUS was inserted under laparoscopic guidance at the time. Antibiotics were given to prevent infection.

Once an IUS or IUCD has been inserted, women should be advised to have their GP check the threads are still visible after the first period. Thereafter most women are willing and able to check the threads themselves.

>   **KEY POINTS**
>
> - The differential diagnosis of lost IUS threads is perforation and migration of the device, expulsion or misplacement of the device within the uterine cavity.
> - Appropriate location at the fundus is essential for full contraceptive efficacy.
> - Women with a 'lost coil' should use alternative contraception.

CASE 33: BLEEDING IN PREGNANCY

History

A 19-year-old woman presents at 13 weeks' gestation with vaginal bleeding and a smelly watery discharge. She feels generally unwell and has had fevers for the last 48 h. She initially thought she had gastroenteritis as she had reduced appetite, abdominal pain, vomiting and loose stools. All her booking bloods were normal and the 11-week 'nuchal' scan was reassuring. She had a previous normal vaginal delivery at 38 weeks' gestation. She has no significant gynaecological or general medical history.

Examination

On examination the temperature is 38.1 degrees, pulse 96/min and blood pressure 110/68 mmHg. She looks flushed and her peripheries are warm. Chest and cardiac examination are normal. She is tender over the uterus, which feels approximately 14 weeks' size. There is no guarding or rebound. On speculum examination the cervical os is closed but an offensive smelling bloodstained discharge is seen. Bimanual examination reveals a very tender and hot uterus that also feels 'boggy'. No adnexal masses are palpable but bilateral adnexal tenderness is evident.

🔍 INVESTIGATIONS

		Normal Range for Pregnancy
Haemoglobin	104 g/L	110–140 g/L
White cell count	24.1 × 10⁹/L	6–16 × 10⁹/L
Neutrophils	18 × 10⁹/L	2.5–7 × 10⁹/L
Platelets	556 × 10⁹/L	150–400 × 10⁹/L
Sodium	135 mmol/L	130–140 mmol/L
Potassium	3.4 mmol/L	3.3–4.1 mmol/L
Urea	6 mmol/L	2.4–4.3 mmol/L
Creatinine	80 mmol/L	34–82 mmol/L
C-reactive protein	127 mg/L	<5 mg/L

Transvaginal ultrasound report: Single intrauterine gestational sac present. Fetus present with crown–rump length 42.7 mm. Fetal heartbeat ABSENT.

The transvaginal ultrasound is shown in Figure 33.1.

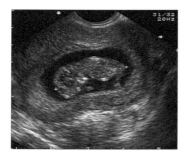

Figure 33.1 Transvaginal ultrasound scan showing a midsagittal view of the uterus.

❓ QUESTIONS

- What is the diagnosis?
- Why is this presentation relatively uncommon in current clinical practice?
- How would you further investigate and manage this woman?

DOI: 10.1201/9781003386933-35

ANSWER 33

The woman is pregnant with a dead fetus and signs of sepsis. This is referred to as a septic miscarriage. This used to be a common diagnosis due to the high incidence of illegal terminations performed by unqualified people without appropriate sterile technique, instruments or anaesthesia. After the 1967 Abortion Act, morbidity and mortality from septic miscarriage fell dramatically but sepsis in early pregnancy remains a cause of maternal mortality, often because it is not recognized early enough. It should therefore be identified promptly and treated aggressively.

Further investigations necessary are blood cultures; liver function tests; coagulation screen, group and save; high vaginal and endocervical swabs.

! COMPLICATIONS OF SEPTIC MISCARRIAGE

- Massive haemorrhage
- Hysterectomy
- Disseminated intravascular coagulopathy
- Multisystem failure (secondary to haemorrhage or sepsis)
- Death

Management

- The woman should be admitted and commenced on broad-spectrum intravenous antibiotics immediately (within 1 hour of attendance) pending culture and sensitivity results.
- Aggressive intravenous fluids should be given as she has intravascular depletion due to sepsis (vasodilatation) and vomiting.
- Surgical evacuation of the uterus should be arranged urgently, once the first dose of antibiotics has been given.
- A senior gynaecologist should be involved as the risks of uterine perforation or of massive haemorrhage are significant in the presence of sepsis.
- A urinary catheter should be inserted to monitor renal function.
- The woman may need transfer to the intensive care unit depending on her cardiovascular, respiratory and haematological state.

🔍 KEY POINTS

- Septic miscarriage is rare since the legalization of termination of pregnancy.
- It should be recognized promptly and treated aggressively due to the risk of rapid deterioration and mortality.
- Complete evacuation of the uterus is essential to eliminate the focus of infection.

CASE 34: PELVIC PAIN

History

A 27-year-old woman complains of left iliac fossa pain. The pain started while she was asleep the night before last and she says it woke her suddenly. Initially the pain was constant and severe and she was unable to get out of bed for a few hours. She felt nauseated and did not eat anything all day yesterday. There was no associated bleeding or discharge and there are no bowel or urinary symptoms. Today the pain is still present but much improved and she has been able to have breakfast.

She has had similar episodes twice in the past but they were not as severe or long lasting. She had never been pregnant and uses the progesterone-only pill (POP) for contraception. She has been with her partner for 3 years and has not had any previous sexually transmitted infections. There is no other medical history of note.

Examination

The temperature is 37.1 degrees, heart rate 76/min and blood pressure 122/70 mmHg. The abdomen is slightly distended and tender in the suprapubic and left iliac fossa regions with some rebound tenderness but no guarding. There are no palpable swellings. Speculum examination is normal and she is tender in the left adnexa on bimanual examination, but no cervical excitation or masses are evident.

🔍 INVESTIGATIONS

		Normal Range
Haemoglobin	123 g/L	117–157 g/L
White cell count	7.1 × 10⁹/L	3.5–11 × 10⁹/L
Platelets	402 × 10⁹/L	150–440 × 10⁹/L
C-reactive protein	2.5 mg/L	<5 mg/L

Urinary pregnancy test: Negative

Urinalysis:
- Protein: Trace
- Blood: Negative
- Leucocytes: Negative
- Nitrites: Negative

Transvaginal ultrasound report: The uterus is anteverted and normal size. The endometrium is thin and measures 3.1 mm. Both ovaries appear normal. There is a moderate amount of anechoic free fluid in the pouch of Douglas, measuring 30 × 26 × 15 mm.

❓ QUESTIONS

- What is the differential diagnosis?
- How would you manage this patient?

DOI: 10.1201/9781003386933-36

ANSWER 34

The sudden onset of left iliac pain suggests rupture, haemorrhage or torsion of an ovarian cyst. In cases of torsion of the ovary this would normally result in vomiting and systemic upset, whereas this woman's condition has in fact improved. In addition in cases of torsion, an adnexal swelling (representing the enlarged oedematous ovary) would be visible on ultrasound. Haemorrhage into a cyst would be seen on transvaginal ultrasound scan as an echogenic ovarian enlargement.

If a cyst ruptures then it is common for the ovary to appear ultrasonographically normal afterwards but the finding of free fluid in the pouch of Douglas supports this pathology.

Thus the diagnosis is likely to be a ruptured ovarian cyst. Alternative diagnoses may include irritable bowel syndrome or possibly renal colic, though urinalysis does not show haematuria.

Management

The patient is already improving and the pelvic free fluid which is causing the peritoneal irritation (and the rebound tenderness) is expected to resolve spontaneously. Therefore immediate management is supportive with analgesia.

In the longer term, the woman should be advised to use a different contraceptive as the POP is known to be associated with an increased incidence of ovarian cysts and it seems from the history that this is the third episode for this woman.

 KEY POINTS

- The only ultrasound evidence of ovarian cyst rupture may be the presence of free peritoneal fluid.
- Ovarian cyst rupture should generally be managed expectantly.
- An increased incidence of ovarian cysts is found in women using the progesterone-only pill, whereas the combined oral contraceptive pill reduces cyst occurrence by inhibiting ovulation.

CASE 35: VULVAL SWELLING

History

A 17-year-old girl presents with a vulval swelling. She noticed a lump a few weeks earlier and in the last 2 days it has enlarged and become painful. She cannot walk normally and has not been able to wear her normal jeans because of the discomfort. She feels well in herself however.

She has been sexually active since the age of 14 years and uses the depot progestogen injection for contraception and therefore does not have periods. She has been with her boyfriend for 8 months and on direct questioning reports unprotected intercourse with two other boys in that time. She had a sexual health screen in a genitourinary clinic 1 year ago and the result was normal. There is no other medical history of note and she takes no medication.

Examination

The temperature is 37.7 degrees, heart rate 68/min and blood pressure normal. Abdominal examination is normal. There is a left-sided posterior labial swelling extending anteriorly from the level of the introitus, measuring $6 \times 4 \times 4$ cm. It appears red, fluctuant, tense and is exquisitely tender to touch. Left-sided tender inguinal lymph nodes are noted.

? | **QUESTIONS**

- What is the diagnosis?
- How would you manage this patient?

DOI: 10.1201/9781003386933-37

ANSWER 35

The diagnosis is of a Bartholin's abscess. The Bartholin glands are located in the posterior vulva and the gland ducts open into the lower vagina to maintain a moist vaginal surface, important during intercourse. Obstruction to a duct by inflammation (from friction during intercourse) or infection causes a cyst to develop, which commonly becomes infected. Usually mixed flora is found but it has been reported that in up to 20 per cent of cases gonorrhoea is isolated.

The diagnosis is clinical and it is important to differentiate a Bartholin's abscess from the differential diagnosis of a sebaceous cyst, vaginal wall cyst or perianal abscess.

Management

The abscess must be drained, traditionally by formal incision and drainage, with the edges of the cyst capsule sutured to the skin to prevent reclosure of the duct (marsupialization).

Increasingly commonly to avoid general anaesthetic, an inflatable balloon catheter ('Word catheter') is inserted into the abscess (or cyst) under local anaesthetic to drain the fluid. This is left for 4 weeks, to allow epithelialization and a long-term drainage route for the gland, thus hopefully reducing the chance of recurrence of the abscess.

In this case, the girl has had several recent partners and a general sexually transmitted infection screen should be arranged after drainage of the cyst, with general sexual health advice.

In most cases antibiotics are not needed after drainage unless there is significant surrounding erythema, systemic signs of sepsis, inguinal lymphadenopathy (as in this case) or gonococcus is found in the culture of the drained fluid.

 KEY POINTS

- Bartholin abscesses are relatively common and cause acute painful unilateral vulval swelling.
- Drainage of the abscess and marsupialization of the skin edges are the mainstay of treatment but recurrence is still common.
- Pus should always be sent for culture as gonorrhoea is isolated from up to 20 per cent of Bartholin abscesses.

CASE 36: ABDOMINAL PAIN

History

A 26-year-old woman presents with abdominal pain. It started suddenly 2 hours ago and was initially in the lower abdomen but is now generalized. She feels nauseated and dizzy, especially when she sits up. She also feels as if she has bruised her shoulder. She has not noticed any vaginal bleeding or discharge, and there are no bowel or urinary symptoms.

She does not keep a record of her period dates but thinks the last one was about a month ago. She has a regular partner and says that they often forget to use a condom.

She had a termination 3 years ago. She was diagnosed with chlamydia when she was admitted to hospital at the age of 19 years with a pelvic infection.

There is no other medical history of note.

Examination

On examination she is pale and looks unwell. She is intermittently drowsy. She is lying flat and still on the bed. The temperature is 35.9 degrees, pulse 120/min and blood pressure 95/50 mmHg. Peripherally she is cool and the hands are clammy. She is generally slim but the abdomen is symmetrically distended. There is generalized tenderness on light palpation, with rebound tenderness and guarding. There are no obviously palpable masses and vaginal examination has not been carried out.

🔍 INVESTIGATIONS

		Normal Range
Haemoglobin	96 g/L	117–157 g/L
Mean cell volume	87 fL	80–99 fL
White cell count	7.1×10^9/L	$3.5–11 \times 10^9$/L
Platelets	204×10^9/L	$150–440 \times 10^9$/L
Sodium	132 mmol/L	135–145 mmol/L
Potassium	6.0 mmol/L	3.5–5 mmol/L
Urea	6 mmol/L	2.5–6.7 mmol/L
Creatinine	70 mmol/L	70–120 mmol/L

Urinary pregnancy test: Positive

❓ QUESTIONS

- What is the likely diagnosis?
- How would you manage the patient?

DOI: 10.1201/9781003386933-38

ANSWER 36

Any woman who is unwell with abdominal pain should be assumed to have a ruptured ectopic pregnancy. In this case there are risk factors and the symptoms of dizziness, nausea, severe abdominal pain and shoulder pain are classical of haemoperitoneum. The examination findings of cool and clammy peripheries, a distended abdomen, tachycardia and hypotension also suggest the clinical diagnosis and a positive pregnancy test confirms this.

Young women tend to compensate for hypovolaemia, and the fact that this woman is now cool and clammy with hypotension suggests that she is gravely unwell and should be transferred for definitive management without delay.

Although the haemoglobin does not seem dramatically reduced, it is likely that on repeat testing it may now be extremely low.

Management

The anaesthetist, theatre staff and senior gynaecologist should be alerted immediately and the woman transferred to theatre for surgery. An ultrasound is not necessary although a focused assessment with sonography for trauma (FAST) scan may show blood in the abdomen and can be carried out quickly in the emergency department. Depending on the haemodynamic status at the time, and on discussion with the anaesthetist, laparoscopy could be considered assuming that the surgeon is very experienced and confident that they can quickly identify and secure a ruptured tube. Alternatively, in an unstable patient laparotomy may still be indicated.

Assuming the diagnosis of tubal rupture was confirmed, then salpingectomy would be necessary (rather than salpingotomy) as the fallopian tube would not be salvageable.

! KEY INITIAL MANAGEMENT FOR SUSPECTED RUPTURED ECTOPIC PREGNANCY

- Facial oxygen
- Lie flat with head down
- Two large-bore cannulae with 2 L of intravenous fluids given immediately
- Crossmatch 4 units (and alert haematologist to the haemorrhage)
- Consent for laparoscopy/laparotomy and salpingectomy
- Transfer to theatre for salpingectomy

Ruptured ectopic pregnancy is still the leading cause of maternal death in early pregnancy, and doctors must be alert to the occasional presentation with life-threatening haemorrhage, as in this case.

 KEY POINTS

- Ectopic pregnancy is still a significant cause of early pregnancy maternal death.
- Any woman of reproductive age who is unwell with abdominal pain and a positive pregnancy test should be assumed to have a ruptured ectopic pregnancy.
- Preoperative ultrasound is not indicated if ectopic pregnancy rupture is suspected.

CASE 37: URINARY RETENTION

History

A 29-year-old woman presents to the emergency department having been unable to pass urine for 8 h. For the last 3 days she has been feeling unwell with a fever, shivering and a reduced appetite. She has pain in her groins specifically but says that her whole body aches. Yesterday she began to feel pain on passing urine, and today this has become very severe such that now she cannot micturate at all. She has never experienced any episodes like this before. She has no previous medical or gynaecology history and has regular menstrual cycles. She recently ended a long-term relationship and has been with a new partner for a few months, with whom she uses condoms.

Examination

The woman is obviously in significant discomfort. Her temperature is 37.4 degrees, heart rate 102/min and blood pressure 118/80 mmHg. Bilateral tender inguinal lymphadenopathy is noted and axillary lymph nodes are also palpable. The bladder is palpable midway to the umbilicus. The vulva is generally reddened and there is a cluster of ulcerated lesions of approximately 2–5 mm on the left side of the labia minora. Speculum examination shows the cervix to be inflamed with a profuse exudate.

INVESTIGATIONS		
		Normal Range
Haemoglobin	127 g/L	117–157 g/L
White cell count	12×10^9/L	$3.5–11 \times 10^9$/L
Neutrophils	3.2×10^9/L	$2–7.5 \times 10^9$/L
Lymphocytes	9×10^9/L	$1.3–3.5 \times 10^9$/L
Platelets	272×10^9/L	$150–440 \times 10^9$/L

QUESTIONS
• What is the diagnosis?
• How would you further investigate and manage this patient?

ANSWER 37

The woman is demonstrating a classic presentation of primary herpes simplex virus infection. Prodromal flu-type symptoms and generalized lymphadenopathy usually occur most significantly with primary infection, whereas any subsequent attacks are more likely to present with vulval soreness as the only noticeable feature.

! HERPES SIMPLEX FEATURES

- *Primary infection:*
  - General malaise
  - Fever
  - Anorexia
  - Lymphadenopathy
  - Genital blisters
  - Urinary retention
- *Recurrent (secondary) infection:*
  - Genital blisters
  - Often occurs at times of stress or tiredness

The woman probably acquired the infection from her new partner – condoms do not effectively prevent infection as the organism can spread from the perineum. In this case there is also evidence of herpes cervicitis from spread of virus particles into the vagina.

Further Investigation

Vulval viral swab should be sent to confirm the diagnosis. This requires firm rubbing of the swab onto an ulcer and is very painful, but as the diagnosis has such profound social implications, confirmation of the diagnosis is imperative.

Management
Immediate Management

- The woman should have an indwelling urinary catheter inserted immediately and be given analgesia and paracetamol.
- Local anaesthetic gel often relieves the pain of the herpes blisters and can be used until symptoms settle.
- Oral aciclovir started within 24 h of an attack reduces the severity and duration of the episode.

Further Management

- Referral to a health counsellor should be made to discuss the diagnosis and its implications.
- Some women have many recurrent attacks, whereas others never experience a further episode. For recurrent attacks aciclovir (or valacyclovir or famciclovir) may be given again if commenced within 24 h of becoming unwell.
- Antiviral suppression treatment is indicated if a woman has recurrent attacks and can reduce the frequency of attacks by 70–80 per cent.
- It is important for women to inform the booking midwife of previous herpes infection at the start of any subsequent pregnancy to ensure prophylactic antiviral treatment can be started appropriately.

🔑 **KEY POINTS**

- Genital herpes simplex infection has a major psychosexual and social impact on sufferers.
- The first attack is generally severe and associated with primarily systemic features.
- Recurrent episodes may be hardly noticed; transmission may occur prior to the appearance of blisters and condoms do not prevent spread of disease and so it is difficult to limit.
- Antiviral treatment does not cure the disease but is effective at reducing the duration and severity of an episode.

CASE 38: ABDOMINAL PAIN

History

A 14-year-old girl presents with lower abdominal pain which developed suddenly a day ago. The pain is over the whole lower abdomen but worse on the right. It was intermittent at first but is now constant and very severe. She feels unwell in herself with no appetite and vomiting. She now feels sweaty as well.

She says her bowels opened normally the day before and they are generally regular.

She has had no previous episodes of pain like this. Her last menstrual period started 2 weeks ago and she has a slightly irregular cycle. She has never had any gynaecological or other medical problems in the past.

Examination

On examination she looks in pain and seems to find it difficult to get comfortable. Her temperature is 37.9 degrees, pulse 112/min and blood pressure 116/74 mmHg. She feels warm and well perfused. The abdomen is distended symmetrically with generalized tenderness, maximal in the right iliac fossa region. There is rebound and guarding in the right iliac fossa.

🔍 INVESTIGATIONS

		Normal Range
Haemoglobin	138 g/L	117–157 g/L
White cell count	14.2 × 10⁹/L	3.5–11 × 10⁹/L
Platelets	390 × 10⁹/L	150–440 × 10⁹/L
C-reactive protein	55 mg/L	<5 mg/L

? QUESTIONS

- What is the differential diagnosis?
- How would you investigate and manage this girl?

ANSWER 38

The differential diagnosis of right iliac fossa pain in this case is:

- *Gynaecological*:
    - Adnexal/ovarian cyst torsion
    - Ovarian cyst rupture
    - Ovarian cyst haemorrhage
    - Ectopic pregnancy
- *Surgical*:
    - Appendicitis
- *Urinary*:
    - Urinary tract infection
    - Renal colic

The girl is acutely systemically unwell with an acute abdomen which would favour the diagnosis of torsion or possibly ruptured appendix. Cyst rupture and haemorrhage are not commonly associated with such systemic disturbance, though this is an important differential diagnosis.

Further investigation would include a pregnancy test to exclude pregnancy, and urinalysis to exclude urinary tract infection or renal colic. An ultrasound should be arranged (transabdominal) to assess for an ovarian cyst or for an inflamed appendix. The ultrasound appearances of adnexal torsion are variable, but there is invariably a unilaterally enlarged oedematous ovary, commonly with a visible cyst or haemorrhage within the ovary. If an adnexal mass is confirmed, laparoscopy should be performed as soon as possible since adnexal torsion is associated with loss of the ovarian function if ischaemia is prolonged and necrosis occurs. Ovarian torsion should be managed with detorsion (ideally laparoscopically) and cystectomy if a large cyst is present. Occasionally, fixing the ovary to the uterus or pelvic side wall to reduce the chance of recurrent torsion would be considered. Only if the ovary is gangrenous is oophorectomy indicated.

If the diagnosis is not clear between appendicitis and ovarian torsion then joint laparoscopy with the surgical team is an appropriate approach.

 KEY POINTS

- Suspected ovarian torsion is a gynaecological emergency.
- Torsion is relatively common in young girls and teenagers.
- Ultrasound is useful in detection of an adnexal mass but torsion is a clinically suspected diagnosis and necessitates urgent laparoscopy.

CASE 39: ABDOMINAL PAIN

History

A 24-year-old student is referred to the gynaecologist on call from the emergency department with sudden onset of left iliac fossa pain which woke her at 2 am. She fell asleep again but since 8 am the pain has been constant and is not relieved by ibuprofen or codydramol.

Her last period started 2 weeks ago and she reports no irregular bleeding or discharge. She has no significant gynaecological history except for a termination of pregnancy at age 17 years. She has been with her current boyfriend for 2 years and has used the combined oral contraceptive pill (COCP) throughout that time. She says she has not had intercourse for the last 4 months because her boyfriend has been travelling, but says that intercourse has never been painful.

On direct questioning she has felt nauseated but has not vomited. She has had no urinary symptoms but has opened her bowels several times each day for the last 3 days, which is unusual for her.

Examination

On examination she is apyrexial, her observations are normal and her abdomen is soft with vague left iliac fossa tenderness but no signs of peritonism. Bimanual examination reveals a normal-sized uterus with no adnexal tenderness or cervical excitation and no obvious adnexal masses.

INVESTIGATIONS

		Normal Range
Haemoglobin	128 g/L	117–157 g/L
Mean cell volume	85 fL	80–99 fL
White cell count	6.4×10^9/L	$3.5–11 \times 10^9$/L
Platelets	178×10^9/L	$150–440 \times 10^9$/L
Sodium	142 mmol/L	135–145 mmol/L
Potassium	3.8 mmol/L	3.5–5 mmol/L
Urea	5.0 mmol/L	2.5–6.7 mmol/L
Creatinine	72 mmol/L	70–120 mmol/L
C-reactive protein	95 mg/L	<5 mg/L

QUESTIONS

- What is the first investigation you would like to perform?
- What is your differential diagnosis if this test is negative, and how would you rule out some of these diagnoses?

DOI: 10.1201/9781003386933-41

ANSWER 39

Any woman of reproductive age with abdominal pain should always have a urinary pregnancy test, regardless of the date of her last menstrual period. In this case the test is negative.

The remaining differential diagnoses include:

- Ovarian cyst
- Pelvic inflammatory disease
- Urinary tract infection or stone
- Bowel-related cause

There are no specific gynaecological symptoms or adnexal tenderness, which implies that the pain is not gynaecological in origin. However during speculum examination it is prudent to send swabs for chlamydia and gonorrhoea infection opportunistically, in view of the high background prevalence of sexually transmitted infection, especially in the 18–25-year-old age group.

Ovulation pain (mittelschmerz) or a corpus luteal cyst are very unlikely as the COCP inhibits the ovulatory cycle. However a transvaginal ultrasound scan will rule out an ovarian cyst for certain.

Urine should be analysed for blood to rule out a renal stone, and for leucocytes and nitrites to rule out infection.

Bowel habit is altered and the raised C-reactive protein suggests an inflammatory condition. As the onset is acute and not severe, the diagnosis is likely to be gastroenteritis. This should be managed expectantly, with fluids, rest and simple analgesia. A stool culture should be sent if the symptoms fail to resolve. Other inflammatory bowel conditions such as Crohn's disease and ulcerative colitis are rare causes to consider if the symptoms are persistent or recurrent.

Irritable bowel syndrome is not associated with raised inflammatory markers, and is therefore not a differential diagnosis in this case.

 KEY POINTS

- Gynaecological, urinary and bowel-related pathology can all be associated with lower abdominal pain.
- A thorough and focused history is always important in making a correct diagnosis.

CASE 40: ABDOMINAL PAIN AND VAGINAL DISCHARGE

History

A 46-year-old woman presents with a month-long history of increasing abdominal pain and a green/yellow vaginal discharge. For the last few days she had been feeling feverish and unwell. The pain is across the lower abdomen but worse on the left. She has no urinary symptoms and has been opening her bowels normally. She has a reduced appetite and mild nausea but has not vomited.

She has had two vaginal deliveries in the past and no other pregnancies. She had a laparotomy about 4 years ago for drainage of a pelvic abscess. Recently she has been under the care of a gynaecologist for heavy and prolonged periods, for which she is taking cyclical norethisterone. There is no other medical or surgical history of note.

Examination

The temperature is 37.8 degrees, pulse 95/min and blood pressure is 136/76 mmHg. The abdomen appears slightly distended and a mass is palpated arising from the pelvis on the left. There is focal tenderness in the left iliac fossa without rebound tenderness or guarding. Speculum examination reveals no discharge or blood, and the cervix appears normal. Cervical excitation and bilateral adnexal tenderness are noted, more marked on the left.

🔍 INVESTIGATIONS

		Normal Range
Haemoglobin	103 g/L	117–157 g/L
Mean cell volume	91 fL	80–99 fL
White cell count	13.8×10^9/L	$3.5–11 \times 10^9$/L
Neutrophils	8.9×10^9/L	$2–7.5 \times 10^9$/L
Platelets	521×10^9/L	$150–440 \times 10^9$/L
C-reactive protein	157 mg/L	<5 mg/L

Transvaginal ultrasound scan report: Ultrasound scan shows a uterus with multiple fibroids. The right ovary appears normal. The left ovary cannot be identified separately from a complex adnexal mass, measuring 7 × 6 × 4 cm (Figure 40.1).

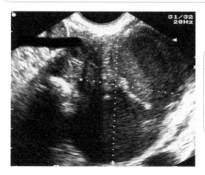

Figure 40.1 Transvaginal ultrasound scan showing the transverse view through the left adnexa.

❓ QUESTIONS

- What is the differential diagnosis?
- Why is she anaemic?
- How would you further investigate and manage this patient?

DOI: 10.1201/9781003386933-42

ANSWER 40

The woman is acutely unwell with pyrexia, tachycardia, raised inflammatory markers, neutrophilia and reactive thrombocythaemia. This suggests an infective process and the left iliac fossa mass detected on ultrasound would appear to be the cause. The likely diagnosis is a tubo-ovarian mass, probably an abscess.

Alternatively this could potentially be a diverticular abscess or, if it were on the right, an appendix abscess. Ovarian malignancy or another cause of a complex adnexal mass would be unlikely to present with this acute inflammatory episode. If there is doubt about the location of the abscess MRI imaging could be considered.

Anaemia in this woman could be due to chronic menorrhagia or anaemia of chronic disease. The increased mean cell volume suggests the latter, but ferritin and folate levels would be useful to see whether there is in fact a degree of iron deficiency, too.

Further Investigation

Blood cultures and vaginal and endocervical swabs should be taken. However in women of this age it is highly unlikely that the infection is due to a newly acquired infection, and is more likely due to anaerobic infection on the background of previous tubal damage.

Ferritin and folate should be checked.

Management

The woman should be admitted for intravenous antibiotics. Broad-spectrum cover should be given including agents against anaerobes and chlamydia. In cases of pelvic inflammatory disease (PID) there is commonly a mixed growth of anaerobes on top of a previous chlamydial infection. If improvement does not occur within 24–48 h, or the diagnosis is unclear, then drainage of the cysts should be considered. This can be carried out transvaginally or transcutaneously, depending on the location of the abscess. If that is not possible then laparoscopy (or laparotomy) should be performed to drain the abscess surgically.

! ADVICE TO PATIENTS WITH PELVIC INFLAMMATORY DISEASE

- The diagnosis (of PID) suggests the likelihood of a sexually transmitted infection either acutely or in the past.
- The partner needs to be screened and treated.
- The couple should avoid intercourse (or use condoms) until both have completed treatment.

🔑 KEY POINTS

- It is common for no organism to be cultured in women with PID.
- A woman with a pelvic abscess due to PID may be given a trial of conservative treatment prior to surgical drainage.
- Contact tracing is an important part of the management of PID to prevent reinfection and further spread of infection.

Section 3
EARLY PREGNANCY

CASE 41: ECTOPIC PREGNANCY MANAGEMENT

History

A 33-year-old woman presents to the early pregnancy unit of the hospital reporting brown vaginal discharge and some mild lower abdominal pain for 2 days. Her last period started 6 weeks 3 days ago and this is her first pregnancy.

Examination

The heart rate is 78/min and blood pressure 115/68 mmHg. The patient appears comfortable. The abdomen is not distended and no masses are palpable. There is no tenderness on palpation.

Speculum examination is normal with no active bleeding seen and the cervix appears normal and closed. No cervical motion tenderness or adnexal tenderness is apparent on bimanual examination.

 INVESTIGATIONS

Urinary pregnancy test: Positive
Transvaginal ultrasound: An empty uterus is noted and a 25 mm swelling is seen adjacent to the left ovary which has the appearance of an ectopic pregnancy. A small gestation sac is seen within the swelling but no embryo or heartbeat is visible. There is no significant free fluid in the pouch of Douglas.
Serum hCG: 4322 IU/L

In view of the high hCG level, medical or expectant management of this ectopic pregnancy would not be appropriate. Laparoscopic surgical management is therefore advised.

? **QUESTIONS**

- Assuming you are the doctor obtaining informed consent for the surgical procedure, how would you counsel the woman regarding whether a salpingectomy or salpingotomy is performed?
- Following surgery what advice should be given to this woman before discharge home?

DOI: 10.1201/9781003386933-44

ANSWER 41

Salpingectomy or Salpingotomy?

Salpingectomy (removal of the fallopian tube with ectopic pregnancy within it) and salpingotomy (linear incision along the antimesenteric border of the tube to remove the ectopic pregnancy) are both reasonable options for this woman, depending on her wishes after full counselling. Although it may seem intuitive to the woman that the tube should not be removed, the following issues should be explained:

1. The risk of persistent trophoblast (due to incomplete removal of all ectopic pregnancy tissue) is 4–8 per cent after salpingotomy but extremely rare after salpingectomy. Therefore there is a small chance of needing methotrexate for a persistently high hCG after salpingotomy.
2. An ectopic pregnancy may suggest a previously poorly functioning tube, prone to recurrent ectopic pregnancy. In addition, the current ectopic pregnancy will have distended the tube and the salpingotomy would damage it further; the risk of subsequent ectopic pregnancy remains higher if the tube is conserved.
3. The risk of repeat ectopic pregnancy after salpingectomy and salpingotomy is approximately 15 and 10 per cent, respectively.
4. The intrauterine pregnancy rate after salpingotomy or salpingectomy is approximately 60 per cent with a nonsignificant trend towards an improved likelihood of subsequent normal intrauterine pregnancy with salpingectomy.
5. At laparoscopy the contralateral tube would be assessed and if it seemed abnormal (blocked or surrounded with adhesions) then all attempts would be made to perform salpingotomy rather than salpingectomy on the tube containing the ectopic pregnancy.
6. It may not be technically possible to perform a salpingotomy and excessive bleeding may necessitate salpingectomy even if salpingectomy is the preferred option preoperatively.

Figures 41.1 and 41.2 show the ultrasound appearance of the ectopic pregnancy and the laparoscopic findings, respectively.

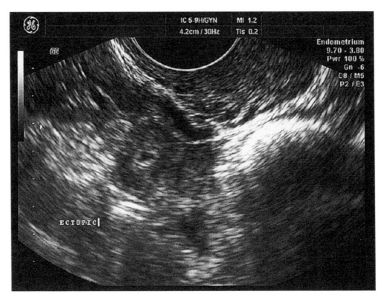

Figure 41.1 Transvaginal ultrasound scan.

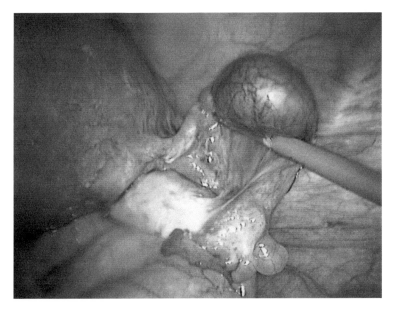

Figure 41.2 Laparoscopy findings.

Advice before Discharge

The box below summarizes the important counselling and advice for a woman following diagnosis of ectopic pregnancy. In addition, if the woman has undergone salpingotomy or there was a suggestion of possible spillage of trophoblast at salpingectomy, then she should have hCG monitoring until the hCG returns to the non-pregnant level (<5 IU/L).

> **! POSTOPERATIVE COUNSELLING POINTS AFTER ECTOPIC PREGNANCY**
>
> - Explanation of diagnosis and proposed operation.
> - Appropriate counselling that the woman may grieve for the loss of the pregnancy, with advice about how to access further support organizations.
> - Advise avoidance, if possible, of the progesterone-only contraceptive pill (POP) and intrauterine contraceptive device (IUCD) (both are associated with a slightly higher risk of ectopic pregnancy).
> - Approximately 60 per cent of women who have had an ectopic pregnancy go on to have a live birth in the next 3 years, but there is a 10–15 per cent chance of a further ectopic pregnancy.
> - Early transvaginal scan is indicated at around 5 weeks' gestation to confirm the location of any future pregnancy.
> - Effective contraception should be used if the woman does not wish to become pregnant again at the moment.

KEY POINTS

- The indications for surgical management of ectopic pregnancy (rather than expectant or medical) are:
  - Haemodynamic instability
  - Live ectopic pregnancy (cardiac activity seen)
  - hCG greater than 3000 IU/L
  - Significant pain
  - Presence of significant haemoperitoneum on ultrasound scan
  - Patient choice/poor compliance with conservative treatment

- The decision to perform a salpingectomy, rather than salpingotomy, depends on patient choice and operative findings.

- hCG follow-up after salpingotomy is essential.

CASE 42: EARLY PREGNANCY ULTRASOUND

History

A 25-year-old woman is referred by the general practitioner (GP) for an early pregnancy dating ultrasound scan. She is gravida 4 para 2. Her first positive pregnancy test was 4 days ago and she went to her GP to arrange a termination of pregnancy as she feels that she cannot cope with another child. She has been taking the combined oral contraceptive pill (COCP), so pregnancy could not be dated clinically. She has no significant gynaecological history of note except for an episode of chlamydia at age 18 years, for which she and her partner were fully treated. As a child she had a ruptured appendix and needed a midline laparotomy. She has no other relevant past medical history.

She has had no pain though did note some moderate vaginal bleeding 2 weeks before for 3 days, which settled spontaneously.

Examination

She looks well with normal heart rate and blood pressure and a soft non-tender abdomen. Speculum examination shows a closed cervix with a normal discharge and no blood. The uterus feels of normal size and is anteverted and mobile. There is no cervical excitation. There is slight tenderness in the left adnexa but no masses are palpable.

🔍 **INVESTIGATIONS**

Transvaginal ultrasound findings are shown in Figure 42.1.

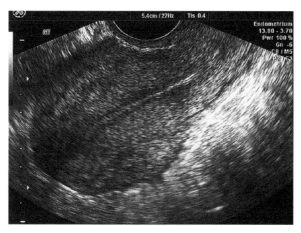

Figure 42.1 Transvaginal ultrasound scan showing a midsagittal view of the uterus.

❓ **QUESTIONS**

- How would you interpret this ultrasound scan result?
- Serial serum human chorionic gonadotrophin (hCG) and progesterone are requested and the results are as follows:
  - Day 1: Serum hCG 703 IU/L, progesterone 30 nmol/L
  - Day 3: Serum hCG 905 IU/L, progesterone 24 nmol/L
- What is the likely diagnosis and the differential diagnosis, and how would you further investigate and manage this woman?

DOI: 10.1201/9781003386933-45

ANSWER 42

The transvaginal ultrasound scan shows an empty uterus and no adnexal masses. This is therefore termed a pregnancy of unknown location (PUL).

> **! DEFINITION OF A PREGNANCY OF UNKNOWN LOCATION**
>
> No ultrasound signs of either intra- or extrauterine pregnancy or retained products of conception in a woman with a positive pregnancy test.

PUL occurs in up to 20 per cent of women in early pregnancy units and the possible underlying diagnoses are:

- Early intrauterine pregnancy which is too early to be visualized on ultrasound.
- Failed pregnancy: A complete miscarriage where the pregnancy has been completely expelled but where no previous scan is available to confirm that an intrauterine pregnancy had been present.
- Ectopic pregnancy where the pregnancy is located outside the uterine cavity but has not been visualized at initial ultrasound examination.

Only 10 per cent of PULs are subsequently diagnosed as ectopic pregnancies, but all must be investigated with serum hCG and progesterone to determine which of the above three diagnoses is likely.

Serum hCG Results and Management

The hCG at which an intrauterine pregnancy would normally be visualized on transvaginal ultrasound scan is 1000–1500 IU/L (in most but not all cases). A normal early pregnancy would generally show an increase in hCG of over 66 per cent in each 48 h. The progesterone level is usually high (>40–60 nmol/L) in an ongoing pregnancy and low (<20 nmol/L) in a failing pregnancy.

In this case, the suboptimal hCG rise and midrange progesterone are typical (but not diagnostic) of an ectopic pregnancy, and the woman should have a repeat ultrasound within a few days. If an ectopic pregnancy is visualized then medical or surgical management should depend on signs and symptoms. If a pregnancy is still not visualized and she becomes symptomatic then laparoscopy is indicated to establish the diagnosis.

> **KEY POINTS**
>
> - Pregnancy of unknown location may represent an early intrauterine pregnancy, a complete miscarriage or an ectopic pregnancy.
> - Follow-up hCG and ultrasound must be arranged for these women.
> - If pain develops before a diagnosis is confirmed, laparoscopy should be carried out to exclude an ectopic pregnancy.

CASE 43: MIDTRIMESTER COMPLICATIONS

History

A 19-year-old woman has attended the emergency department with vaginal discharge. She is 17 weeks' gestation in her third pregnancy. The previous two pregnancies were terminated medically in the first trimester using prostaglandins. This pregnancy was unplanned but she is now looking forward to being a mother.

She had a small amount of bleeding at around 7 weeks, which persisted until 9 weeks. Ultrasound scan at 7 weeks showed a single live embryo.

She booked for antenatal care late at 13 weeks. The combined test for Down's syndrome showed low risk (1:5100).

She is a non-smoker and has drunk no alcohol since finding out she was pregnant at 7 weeks. She has no other significant medical history.

On direct questioning the vaginal loss started a few hours ago. Initially she thought it was possibly urine that was leaking but it has no smell and she is sure it is now coming from the vagina. There has been a minimal amount of blood on the pad but it is mainly clear fluid. Initially the fluid soaked through all of her clothes, but it is now less. There has been no abdominal pain.

Examination

She appears distressed. Her temperature is 37.1 degrees, blood pressure is 115/68 mmHg and pulse is 84/min.

Abdominally the uterus is palpable about one-third of the way between pubic symphysis and umbilicus and feels soft. The abdomen is non-tender.

Speculum examination shows the cervix to appear normal and closed. There is a moderate amount of clear watery shiny fluid pooling in the speculum, which is also seen coming from the cervix when the woman is asked to cough.

🔍 **INVESTIGATIONS**

		Normal Range for Pregnancy
Haemoglobin	108 g/L	110–140 g/L
Mean cell volume	92 fL	74.4–95.6 fL
White cell count	6.9×10^9/L	$6–16 \times 10^9$/L
Platelets	321×10^9/L	$150–400 \times 10^9$/L
C-reactive protein	11.3 mg/L	<10 mg/L

Urinalysis: Trace protein; no leucocytes; no nitrites

❓ **QUESTIONS**

- What is the diagnosis?
- What is the prognosis and what should you say to the woman?
- What, if any, further investigations should be requested and what would be your management plan?

DOI: 10.1201/9781003386933-46

ANSWER 43

Diagnosis

The history and speculum findings are very highly suggestive of rupture of membranes at 17 weeks' gestation. This is relatively rare but the presence of persistent first-trimester bleeding is a risk factor, probably because the blood and haemosiderin cause irritation and ultimately necrotic breakdown of the membranes. The other likely cause is subclinical infection. Bacterial vaginosis in particular is associated with increased risk of midtrimester fetal loss.

! PROGNOSIS AND COMMUNICATION TO THE WOMAN

The prognosis in such cases of premature rupture of membranes is extremely poor. This is because of the various complications that may develop as a result:

1. Spontaneous miscarriage is common after rupture of membranes.
2. Chorioamnionitis is likely to develop once the integrity of the gestation sac has been breached.
3. If miscarriage or infection does not occur, then the fetus is likely to have profound pulmonary hypoplasia due to lack of amniotic fluid, as well as limb contractures.

The woman must be offered a grave prognosis for the pregnancy, with respect to not only the chance of fetal survival but also the chance of her developing chorioamnionitis, the onset of which can be sudden and catastrophic.

Further Investigation and Management

To confirm the diagnosis and to check whether the fetal heartbeat is still present an ultrasound scan should be performed. If the fetus has died then medical evacuation of the pregnancy should be carried out without delay.

If the fetus is alive and the scan confirms anhydramnios or oligohydramnios then the woman should be given the option of termination of the pregnancy. This would be in her best interests in terms of preventing serious maternal infection. In view of the poor prognosis for the fetus, many women would choose this option.

If she declines termination then she should be closely monitored for symptoms and signs of infection such as fever, shivering, flu-type symptoms, abdominal pain, offensive vaginal discharge or bleeding. Pyrexia >37.5 degrees, tachycardia, hypotension or increased respiratory rate should be looked for. Alternate-day serum C-reactive protein and white cell count should be checked. There should be a very low threshold for recommending termination of the pregnancy if any combination of these features develops, as sepsis is a leading cause of maternal death in the UK, with one-third of such deaths occurring before 24 weeks' gestation.

Whether the pregnancy is terminated due to fetal death, maternal choice or maternal infection, the first-line method would be the use of prostaglandin, preceded by mifepristone (a progesterone antagonist) 48 hours earlier if time allows.

> 🔑 **KEY POINTS**
>
> - The prognosis for a baby after rupture of membranes in the second trimester is extremely poor.
> - The risks of sepsis and its consequences for the mother should be considered as very important in counselling the woman regarding continuation of the pregnancy after second-trimester rupture of membranes.
> - The woman should be advised to report any symptoms or signs of possible sepsis and these should be acted on as soon as possible.

CASE 44: PAIN AND BLEEDING IN EARLY PREGNANCY

History

A 30-year-old woman is referred from her GP. She is 11 weeks and 2 days' gestation and has noticed dark spotting and mild period-like pains for the last 4 days. Her last period was 4 months ago but she has a history of polycystic ovarian syndrome and has an irregular cycle, bleeding for between 4 and 7 days every 5–6 weeks. She had a positive home pregnancy test after she noticed breast tenderness, and came for a dating ultrasound scan 4 weeks ago that confirmed a correctly sited single live pregnancy. Since then she has had a booking visit with the midwife and all routine blood tests are normal. She is gravida 2 para 0. Her last pregnancy 9 months ago ended in a complete miscarriage at 7 weeks. There is no other medical or gynaecological history of significance.

Examination

She is apyrexial with normal heart rate and blood pressure. The abdomen is soft and non-tender. Speculum examination shows a small cervical ectropion but this is not bleeding. The cervix appears closed and no blood or abnormal discharge is seen. Bimanual examination reveals an 8–10-week-sized anteverted mobile uterus with no cervical motion tenderness or adnexal masses.

🔍 **INVESTIGATIONS**

Transvaginal ultrasound scan report (Figure 44.1): The uterus contains a gestational sac measuring 49 × 48 × 36 mm. A single fetus of crown–rump length 47 mm is visible. Fetal heartbeat is absent. The uterus is anteverted. Both ovaries appear normal with no adnexal masses visible.

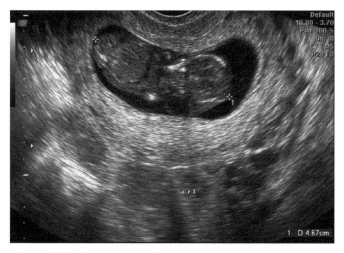

Figure 44.1 Transvaginal ultrasound scan showing the mid-sagittal view through the uterus.

❓ **QUESTIONS**

- What is the diagnosis?
- How would you investigate and manage this patient?

DOI: 10.1201/9781003386933-47

ANSWER 44

The diagnosis is of early embryonic demise (also known as a missed miscarriage). Alternative terminologies for this condition are delayed miscarriage or silent miscarriage.

The diagnosis can be made for two reasons. First, the fetal heartbeat has been seen previously and is no longer visible. Second, where the crown–rump length exceeds 7 mm, a fetal heartbeat should be visible on transvaginal ultrasound in all cases of a live pregnancy. Thus the diagnosis could have been made even if the previous scan result was not known.

The term 'empty sac' (blighted ovum or anembyonic pregnancy) is used where the pregnancy has failed at a much earlier stage, such that the embryo did not become large enough to be visualized, but a sac is still seen. The diagnosis of an empty gestational sac miscarriage can be made when the mean sac diameter exceeds 25 mm with no visible embryo or fetus. This is illustrated in Figure 44.2. The management of early embryonic demise and empty sac miscarriage is the same.

Management

The woman needs to discuss how to proceed now and also what has happened and what she might expect for future pregnancies. The management of miscarriage is expectant, medical or surgical. The choice should be given with the potential advantages and disadvantages of each:

- *Expectant ('wait-and-see') approach*:
    - Avoids medical intervention and can usually be managed completely at home.
    - May involve significant pain and bleeding.
    - Unpredictable time frame – the miscarriage may even take several weeks.
    - More successful for incomplete miscarriage than for missed miscarriage.

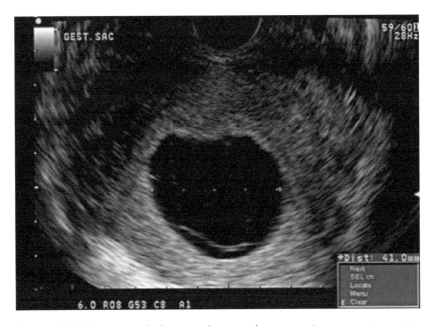

Figure 44.2 Transvaginal ultrasound image demonstrating an empty gestational sac with mean sac diameter greater than 25 mm, confirming the diagnosis of miscarriage.

- *Medical (intravaginal or oral misoprostol tablets, sometimes preceded by mifepristone)*:
  - Similar approach to expectant but more predictable (the miscarriage usually begins within 6–8 hours of the insertion of tablets).
  - Avoids surgical intervention and general anaesthetic.
  - The woman may retain some feeling of being in control.
  - Equivalent infection and bleeding rate as for surgical management (2–3 per cent).
  - Surgical evacuation may be indicated if medical management fails.
- *Surgical (evacuation of retained products of conception)*:
  - Can be arranged within a few days and avoids prolonged follow-up.
  - Very low rate of failure (retained products of conception).
  - Small risk of uterine perforation or anaesthetic complication.

Success rates for missed miscarriage are usually higher for medical or surgical management, whereas expectant management is very successful for incomplete miscarriage.

! IMPORTANT COUNSELLING POINTS AFTER MISCARRIAGE

- Express sympathy – this is a very significant event for the couple and they may perceive the pregnancy loss as strongly as they would the loss of a full-term baby.
- Offer further counselling if needed and give written advice sheets/leaflets.
- Reassure that the miscarriage would not have been a result of anything she has done, such as lifting heavy objects, having a glass of alcohol or having sexual intercourse (all common reasons for women to feel they may be responsible for the loss).
- Explain that over 60 per cent of early pregnancy losses are due to sporadic chromosomal abnormalities such as trisomies, which cannot be avoided.
- Explain that although she has had two consecutive early pregnancy losses there is still a high chance (>70 per cent) that she will have a normal pregnancy in the future.

Further investigation into recurrent miscarriage is usually reserved for those with three or more consecutive losses, because miscarriage is extremely common and even those couples with two miscarriages are extremely unlikely to have any underlying cause for their pregnancy losses.

 KEY POINTS

- Most miscarriages are due to sporadic fetal chromosomal abnormalities.
- A miscarriage may be managed expectantly, medically or surgically.
- Never forget that a miscarriage may be a significant life event for a woman/couple, regardless of whether or not the pregnancy was planned.

CASE 45: BLEEDING IN EARLY PREGNANCY

History

A 36-year-old woman presents with vaginal bleeding at 8 weeks 3 days' gestation. She has never been pregnant before. Bright red 'spotting' commenced 7 days ago, which she thought was normal in early pregnancy. However since then the bleeding is now almost as heavy as a period. There are no clots. She has no abdominal pain. Systemically she has felt nausea for 3 weeks and has vomited occasionally. She had large-loop excision of the transformation zone (LLETZ) treatment after an abnormal smear 6 years ago. Since then, all smears have been normal. There is no other significant gynaecological history. She has regular periods, bleeding for 5 days every 28 days, and has never had any known sexually transmitted infections. In the past she used condoms for contraception.

Examination

The heart rate is 68/min and blood pressure is 108/70 mmHg. The abdomen is soft and non-tender. Speculum reveals a normal closed cervix with a small amount of fresh blood coming from the cervical canal. Bimanually the uterus feels bulky and soft, approximately 10 weeks in size. There is no cervical excitation or adnexal tenderness.

 INVESTIGATIONS

Urinary pregnancy test: Positive

Figure 45.1 shows the transvaginal ultrasound findings.

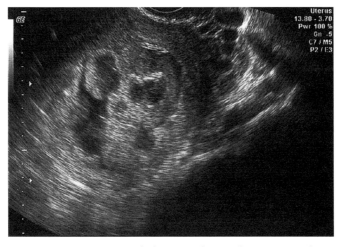

Figure 45.1 Transvaginal ultrasound scan showing a midsagittal view through the uterus.

? **QUESTIONS**

- What is the likely diagnosis and differential diagnosis?
- What would one expect to see at scan in this woman if the pregnancy was normal?
- How would you manage the patient?

DOI: 10.1201/9781003386933-48

ANSWER 45

The ultrasound scan shows a mixed echogenicity appearance in the uterus, typical of a complete hydatidiform mole (molar pregnancy, part of the spectrum of gestational trophoblastic disease). There is no recognizable gestational sac or embryo.

This appearance may also be seen occasionally in pregnancies where early embryonic demise has occurred but the sac has not been expelled (delayed miscarriage) resulting in cystic degeneration of the placenta.

The incidence of molar pregnancy (also known as gestational trophoblastic disease) is approximately 1 in 714. It generally presents with painless vaginal bleeding though it may be diagnosed as an incidental finding when ultrasound is performed for another indication. The classical associations with hyperemesis, thyrotoxicosis or pre-eclampsia are rarely seen in the developed world where diagnosis is generally made in the first trimester.

Normal Findings at 8 Weeks

The normal findings at 8 weeks would be an embryo of approximately 18 mm, with a visible heartbeat. The yolk sac would still be visible and the amniotic sac would also be seen. The embryo would be beginning to develop visible arm and limb buds and embryonic movement may be seen.

Figure 45.2 shows a transvaginal image of a normal 8-week gestation sac and embryo.

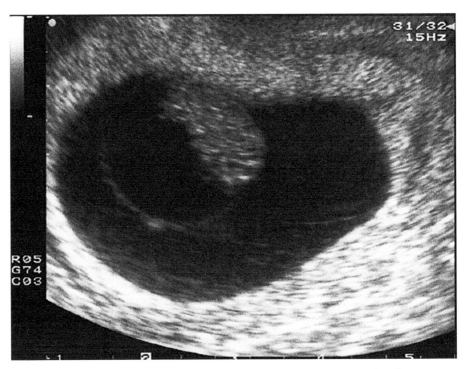

Figure 45.2 Transvaginal image of a normal 8-week gestation sac and embryo (amniotic sac is seen but yolk sac is not visible in this view).

Further Management

The management for suspected molar pregnancy is always surgical evacuation of the uterus, with urgent histological examination of the tissue.

Once diagnosis is confirmed by histology, any woman with a confirmed partial or complete molar pregnancy should be referred to a specialist gestational trophoblastic disease centre (in the UK in Sheffield, Dundee and Charing Cross Hospital) for follow-up of human chorionic gonadotrophin (hCG) levels. Women with persistently raised hCG levels are offered chemotherapy to destroy the persistent trophoblastic tissue and minimize the chance of development of choriocarcinoma. Only 0.5 per cent of women diagnosed with a partial molar pregnancy will require chemotherapy, compared with 10–15 per cent of women with a complete molar pregnancy. Those requiring chemotherapy should not conceive for 1 year after completion of treatment.

Most women, however, do not require chemotherapy as the hCG becomes negative within a short period of time. These women should be advised:

- Not to become pregnant again until the hCG is normal.
- There is a 1 in 84 chance of a further molar pregnancy.
- The combined oral contraceptive pill may safely be used once hCG has returned to normal.

In order to rule out gestational trophoblastic disease in women who do not have histological analysis of the pregnancy tissue, it is recommended that women with early pregnancy loss (miscarriage or ectopic pregnancy) do a urine pregnancy test 3 weeks following any management and contact their Early Pregnancy Unit if still positive.

 KEY POINTS

- Molar pregnancy may be suspected on ultrasound examination but the diagnosis must be confirmed with histological examination of products of conception after surgical uterine evacuation.
- Molar pregnancies must be followed up at a specialist gestational trophoblastic disease centre.
- Development of choriocarcinoma after molar pregnancy is rare, but persistent trophoblastic disease requiring chemotherapy is more common.

CASE 46: BLEEDING IN EARLY PREGNANCY

History

A 31-year-old woman presents with vaginal bleeding at 5 weeks 6 days' gestation. She has had a previous left uterine tubal ectopic pregnancy managed with laparoscopic salpingectomy. She is certain of her last menstrual period date and has regular cycles. Her last smear test was normal and she has not used contraception since her last pregnancy 3 years ago.

When she was 21 years she had an episode of pelvic inflammatory disease treated with intravenous antibiotics. She is otherwise not aware of having had any sexually transmitted infections. She has been with her partner for 7 years. She smokes 10 cigarettes per day and does not drink alcohol. The bleeding is described as very light and she has not been aware of any pain. She has not felt dizzy or lightheaded and has no shoulder-tip pain.

Examination

She is warm and well perfused. The blood pressure is 136/78 mmHg and heart rate 75/min. The abdomen is not distended and no tenderness is elicited on palpation. The cervix is closed. The uterus feels normal size, anteverted and mobile, and there is no cervical motion tenderness. Gentle adnexal examination shows no significant tenderness.

 INVESTIGATIONS

Human chorionic gonadotrophin (β-hCG): 691 IU/L

Transvaginal ultrasound scan findings are shown in Figures 46.1 and 46.2.

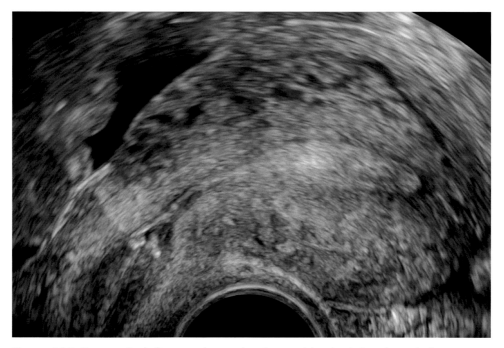

Figure 46.1 Transvaginal ultrasound scan showing a midsagittal view through the uterus.

DOI: 10.1201/9781003386933-49

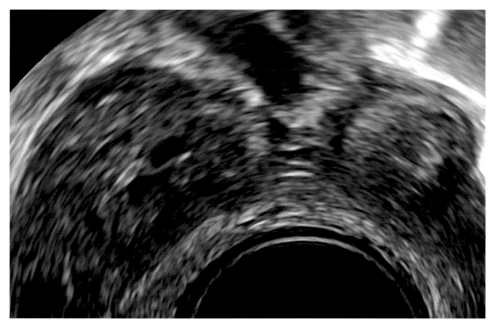

Figure 46.2 Transvaginal ultrasound scan showing a transverse view through the right adnexa.

? **QUESTIONS**

- What is the diagnosis?
- What management options are available and which management would be preferred in this particular case?

ANSWER 46

The ultrasound scan images show an empty uterus and an adnexal swelling adjacent to the right ovary. The swelling represents an ectopic pregnancy. No gestation sac or embryo is visible. However, there is still a possibility of tubal rupture if not treated.

! RISK FACTORS FOR ECTOPIC PREGNANCY

- Smoking
- Previous pelvic inflammatory disease or chlamydial infection
- History of infertility
- *In vitro* fertilization
- Previous tubal surgery
- Previous ectopic pregnancy
- Intrauterine contraceptive device (IUCD) or progesterone-only pill

---

Management

Three options might be appropriate to this woman:

- *Surgical*: Laparoscopic excision of the tube (salpingectomy) or salpingotomy to incise the tube and flush out the ectopic pregnancy.
- *Medical*: Intramuscular methotrexate to destroy the rapidly dividing trophoblast tissue, with regular hCG follow-up to confirm resolution. As methotrexate is teratogenic, it should be given only once a possible intrauterine pregnancy has been completely ruled out. In this case, this may be by repeat hCG in 48 h to be certain that the change is not consistent with a potentially live pregnancy.
- *Expectant*: 'Wait-and-see' approach, suitable if the hCG is decreasing spontaneously when repeated after 48 hours and the woman remains asymptomatic.

In this case, the woman has previously had a uterine tube removed and surgery might compromise the remaining tube, so methotrexate treatment is preferred. However if the tube is damaged but preserved, she may be at high risk of further ectopic pregnancy. Prerequisites for methotrexate are normal full blood count, renal and liver function before treatment, compliance with the intense follow-up and understanding the need not to become pregnant again for at least 3 months due to the potential teratogenic effects. Potential side effects of methotrexate are abdominal pain (sometimes difficult to distinguish from pain suggestive of tubal rupture), nausea, diarrhoea and, rarely, conjunctivitis and stomatitis.

  KEY POINTS

- Ectopic pregnancies are commonly asymptomatic or associated with atypical symptoms.
- Surgical, medical or expectant management of ectopic pregnancy depends on the symptoms, signs and hCG result.
- Methotrexate is effective but follow-up is intensive and sometimes prolonged.
- Methotrexate should never be administered if there is a possibility of a potentially viable intrauterine pregnancy.

CASE 47: BLEEDING IN EARLY PREGNANCY

History

A 41-year-old woman is seen in the early pregnancy unit because of vaginal bleeding. She is gravida 4 para 2 having had two previous normal vaginal deliveries followed by a miscarriage. She has a regular 28-day menstrual cycle and her last period started 9 weeks ago. She had slight vaginal bleeding 2 weeks ago and on ultrasound scan an early intrauterine pregnancy had been visualized with gestational sac of $18 \times 12 \times 22$ mm diameter and a yolk sac visualized of $4 \times 5 \times 5$ mm. No embryo was visualized. She was given an appointment for a repeat ultrasound.

Four days ago her bleeding became very heavy and she passed large clots which she described as 'like liver'. She developed severe abdominal pain which lasted for about 4 h, and since then the bleeding has become very light and she is now pain-free.

She has normal appetite and no nausea or vomiting. She has no urinary or bowel symptoms.

Examination

She appears well and is apyrexial. There are no signs of anaemia. The heart rate is 82/min and blood pressure is 132/78 mmHg. The abdomen is soft and mildly tender suprapubically. Speculum shows the cervix is closed with a small amount of old blood in the vagina. There is slight uterine tenderness on bimanual palpation and the uterus feels normal size, anteverted and mobile, with no adnexal tenderness or cervical motion tenderness.

🔍 **INVESTIGATIONS**

A transvaginal ultrasound scan is shown in Figure 47.1.

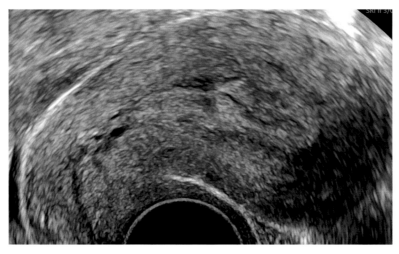

Figure 47.1 Transvaginal ultrasound scan showing a midsagittal view through the uterus.

❓ **QUESTIONS**

- What is the diagnosis?
- What further management is indicated?

DOI: 10.1201/9781003386933-50

ANSWER 47

The ultrasound image shows a longitudinal view of the uterus. There is a small amount of blood within the cavity and the endometrium is disrupted. There is no visible gestation sac or retained products of conception. As we know from the previous report that there was previously an intra-uterine pregnancy, we can conclude that this is a complete miscarriage. If a previous ultrasound had not been available we would need to treat the case as a pregnancy of unknown location and monitor serial serum hCG and progesterone.

No further management is needed as the miscarriage is complete and there are no signs of retained products of conception, or any suggestion of sepsis. Anti-D is not needed even if the woman is rhesus negative as the pregnancy is less than 12 weeks' gestation.

Counselling is the most important part of this consultation, as explained in Case 44.

There is no clear evidence that a longer interpregnancy interval improves the outcome in future pregnancies, and the couple should be informed that they may try and conceive whenever they choose. However, it may be advisable to wait until after the next menstrual period (usually 4–6 weeks after a miscarriage) in order to date the pregnancy.

Reassurance scans are helpful in future pregnancies and may improve outcome. In view of the two consecutive losses, reassurance ultrasound at 7 weeks and then at intervals until the 11–14-week scan would be ideal.

 KEY POINTS

- Clinical suspicion alone is not sufficient to make a diagnosis of miscarriage.
- If the uterus is empty and an intrauterine gestation has not been previously confirmed then a case should be treated as a pregnancy of unknown location, with serum hCG and progesterone to guide follow-up.
- Appropriate counselling is vital in the management of couples with early pregnancy loss.

CASE 48: VOMITING IN PREGNANCY

History

A 28-year-old Asian woman is referred by her GP with persistent vomiting at 7 weeks' gestation. She is in her second pregnancy having had a normal vaginal delivery 3 years ago. She is now vomiting up to 10 times in 24 h, and has not managed to tolerate any food for 3 days. She can only drink small amounts of water.

She saw her GP a week ago who prescribed oral prochlorperazine but these only helped for a few days. She feels very weak in herself and is unable to care for her son now.

On direct questioning she has upper abdominal pain that is constant, sharp and burning. She has not opened her bowels for 5 days. She is passing small amounts of dark urine infrequently but there is no dysuria or haematuria. There has been no vaginal bleeding.

There is no other medical or gynaecological history of note except that she suffered persistent vomiting in her first pregnancy requiring two overnight admissions.

Examination

She is apyrexial. Lying blood pressure is 115/68 mmHg and standing blood pressure 98/55 mmHg. Heart rate is 96/min. The mucus membranes appear dry. Abdominal examination reveals tenderness in the epigastrium but no lower abdominal tenderness. The uterus is not palpable abdominally.

INVESTIGATIONS

		Normal Range for Pregnancy
Haemoglobin	111 g/L	110–140 g/L
Mean cell volume	90 fL	74.4–95 fL
White cell count	8.9×10^9/L	6–16×10^9/L
Platelets	298×10^9/L	150–400×10^9/L
Sodium	131 mmol/L	130–140 mmol/L
Potassium	3.0 mmol/L	3.3–4.1 mmol/L
Urea	8.2 mmol/L	2.4–4.3 mmol/L
Creatinine	65 mmol/L	34–82 mmol/L
Alanine transaminase	30 IU/L	6–32 IU/L
Alkaline phosphatase	276 IU/L	30–300 IU/L
Gamma glutamyl transaminase	17 IU/L	5–43 IU/L
Bilirubin	12 mmol/L	3–14 mmol/L
Albumin	34 g/L	28–37 g/L

- Pregnancy test: Positive
- Urinalysis: Protein negative; blood negative; nitrites negative; leucocytes negative; ketones ++++; glucose negative

QUESTIONS

- What is the diagnosis?
- What are the potential complications of this disorder?
- How would you further investigate and manage this patient?

DOI: 10.1201/9781003386933-51

ANSWER 48

The woman is suffering from hyperemesis gravidarum. This affects less than 2 per cent of pregnancies, although more than 50 per cent of women report some nausea or vomiting when pregnant. Hyperemesis gravidarum can be diagnosed when there is protracted nausea and vomiting with the triad of more than 5 per cent prepregnancy weight loss, dehydration and electrolyte imbalance.

! DIFFERENTIAL DIAGNOSIS OF VOMITING IN EARLY PREGNANCY

- Urinary tract infection
- Gastroenteritis
- Thyrotoxicosis
- Hepatitis

The diagnosis in this case can be made after excluding other causes of her symptoms; the urinalysis is negative apart from the ketones, so urinary tract infection is very unlikely. She has not opened her bowels but this is likely to be secondary to poor dietary intake and dehydration. Liver function is normal, so liver disease causing vomiting is unlikely (though abnormal liver function may occur as a result of hyperemesis itself). Thyroid function is normal, so an alternative diagnosis of hyperthyroidism causing the vomiting is unlikely.

! COMPLICATIONS OF HYPEREMESIS GRAVIDARUM

- Wernicke's encephalopathy (from vitamin B deficiency)
- Korsakoff's syndrome (from vitamin B deficiency)
- Haematemesis (from Mallory–Weiss tear)
- Psychological – resentment towards the pregnancy and expression of desire to terminate the pregnancy

---

The fetus is not at risk from hyperemesis and the nutritional deficiency in the mother generally does not seem to affect development in the first trimester. The risk of miscarriage is lower in women with hyperemesis. The risk of twins and molar pregnancy has traditionally been thought to be greater in women with hyperemesis, but this is refuted in more recent research.

Further Investigation and Management

Hyperemesis is a self-limiting disease and the aim of treatments is supportive, with discharge of the woman once she is tolerating food and drink.

Fluids: 3–4 L of normal saline should be infused per day. Dextrose solutions are contraindicated as they may precipitate Wernicke's encephaolopathy and also because the woman is hyponatraemic and needs normal saline.

Potassium: Excessive vomiting generally leads to hypokalaemia, as in this case, and potassium chloride should be administered with the normal saline according to the serum electrolyte results.

Antiemetics: First-line antiemetics include cyclizine (antihistamine), metoclopramide (dopamine antagonist) or prochlorperazine (phenothiazine). A doxylamine/pyridoxine combination was recently licensed for use in nausea and vomiting of pregnancy. In severe cases, ondansetron may be effective. There is poor evidence that ondansetron is associated with development of cleft palate in the fetus and the patient should be counselled on this prior to administration.

Thiamine and folic acid: Vitamin B₁ (thiamine) can prevent Wernicke's encephalopathy or the irreversible Korsakoff's syndrome (amnesia, confabulation, impaired learning ability).

Antacids: For epigastric pain.

Steroids: Steroids can be used in refractory cases of hyperemesis but again the patient must be counselled about the possible impacts of these on the fetus.

Total parenteral nutrition (TPN): TPN is rarely indicated but may be life saving where all other management strategies have failed.

Thromboembolic stockings (TEDS) and heparin: Women with hyperemesis are at risk of thrombosis from pregnancy, immobility and dehydration, and should be considered for low-molecular-weight heparin regime as well as TEDS.

Monitoring

Daily monitoring should be carried out with weight measurement and urinalysis for ketones and renal and liver function.

 KEY POINTS

- Hyperemesis gravidarum is a diagnosis of exclusion.
- There is generally no adverse effect on the fetus in the first trimester.
- Treatment is supportive.
- Thiamine replacement prevents Wernicke's encephalopathy and Korsakoff's syndrome.

Section 4
GENERAL OBSTETRICS

CASE 49: PAIN IN PREGNANCY

History

A 33-year-old Asian woman complains of worsening abdominal pain for 4 days. She is 16 weeks pregnant in her third pregnancy. She has a 10-year-old son by normal delivery, and had a miscarriage 8 years ago. Her pregnancy has been uneventful until now with an unremarkable first-trimester scan.

The pain is in the left lower abdomen and is constant and sharp. She has taken paracetamol with little effect and she is unable to sleep due to the pain.

She has had no vaginal bleeding and reports urinary frequency since the beginning of the pregnancy. She is mildly constipated and has no nausea and vomiting. There is no history of trauma. She has not yet felt the baby moving.

Examination

The woman is apyrexial and pulse rate is 125/min, with blood pressure 110/68 mmHg. The uterus is palpable just above the umbilicus. There is significant tenderness over the left uterine fundal region, where it also feels firm. The abdomen is otherwise soft and non-tender. There is voluntary guarding but no rebound tenderness. Bowel sounds are normal. Speculum examination shows a normal, closed cervix and no blood. The fetal heartbeat is heard with hand-held fetal Doppler.

INVESTIGATIONS		
		Normal Range for Pregnancy
Haemoglobin	106 g/L	110–140 g/L
Mean cell volume	79 fL	74.4–95.6 fL
White cell count	7.2×10^9/L	$6–16 \times 10^9$/L
Platelets	378×10^9/L	$150–400 \times 10^9$/L
C-reactive protein	5 mg/L	<10 mg/L

? QUESTIONS

- What is the likely diagnosis and how should it be confirmed?
- How would you manage this woman?
- What effect will this condition have on the pregnancy?

DOI: 10.1201/9781003386933-53

ANSWER 49

The diagnosis is of fibroid degeneration. The uterine size larger than dates and the localized uterine tenderness are the important features in making this diagnosis. Fibroids affect 20–30 per cent of the female population, commonly developing between 30 and 50 years. They are particularly common in African-Caribbean women.

Fibroids are oestrogen sensitive and therefore grow in pregnancy in response to the hyperoestrogenic state. When they outgrow their blood supply they undergo 'red degeneration', with necrosis within the fibroid causing the intense localized pain. The diagnosis of fibroids is confirmed by ultrasound visualization of an encapsulated mass in the uterus. The degeneration is confirmed by the ultrasound appearance of cystic spaces within the fibroid mass.

Degeneration pain usually starts gradually, and some women manage at home with simple paracetamol and rest until the pain subsides. However it is common for the pain to be severe enough for admission to hospital for opiate analgesia. Opiates are safe in pregnancy provided use is not prolonged. Intravenous fluids may be required if the woman is not drinking, or is vomiting due to the pain.

Most women remain well systemically, although a full blood count and C-reactive protein should be taken to check haemoglobin and to assess the white blood count and inflammatory markers. In this case the woman has a mild microcytic anaemia of pregnancy and should be given ferrous sulphate.

The pregnancy itself is not usually compromised by degenerating fibroids except in the rare cases where sepsis develops, in which case miscarriage may occur.

Fibroids are managed expectantly in pregnancy but may cause malpresentation at term, or obstructed labour if there is a pelvic fibroid. In either of these circumstances, caesarean section should be performed. Fibroids are also an independent risk factor for postpartum haemorrhage as they can prevent effective contraction of the uterus after delivery of the placenta. Most fibroids shrink spontaneously during the puerperium, so consideration of surgery should be deferred for at least 3 months after delivery.

 KEY POINTS

- Fibroids are common and may cause pain as they outgrow their blood supply and undergo 'red degeneration'.
- The pain is self-limiting and treatment is pain management.

CASE 50: ILLEGAL DRUG USE IN PREGNANCY

History

A 19-year-old woman is referred to the antenatal clinic by her general practitioner. She is currently 22 weeks' gestation in her second pregnancy. She had a son by normal vaginal delivery 18 months ago, who was taken into social services care initially and now lives with his grandparents (the father's parents). Since then, the woman has been having very infrequent periods and only discovered she was pregnant when she attended the emergency department with a presumed urinary tract infection 2 weeks ago. At that stage abdominal palpation revealed a mass, and ultrasound scan confirmed the single gestation.

The GP letter informs that the woman has been a user of crack cocaine and heroin in the past but that she has been on a methadone replacement programme for the last 8 weeks. The current prescribed regime is 60 mL methadone, which she collects daily from the pharmacist.

The woman reports that she still injects street heroin several times per week but has not used crack cocaine for several months. She says that she drinks minimal alcohol but she smokes 20–25 cigarettes per day.

There is no other medical history of note.

She lives in a council flat with her partner who is also taking prescribed methadone. She denies any domestic violence within the relationship.

Examination

The woman appears thin and anxious. The blood pressure is 107/65 mmHg and pulse 90/min. The abdomen is distended with the fundus palpable at the umbilicus. The fetal heartbeat is heard with a hand-held Doppler device.

INVESTIGATIONS

Rubella: Immune
Syphilis: Negative
Hepatitis B surface antigen: Positive
HIV1/2: Negative
Haemoglobin: 114 g/L
Blood group: A positive

? QUESTIONS

- What other investigations should be arranged?
- What are the risks associated with drug use in pregnancy?
- How would you manage this woman during the pregnancy?

ANSWER 50

The woman has been found to be hepatitis B surface antigen positive. This needs further investigation with e antigenicity to determine risk of transmission, and liver function tests. Assuming the hepatitis B is related to needle sharing, she is also at significant risk of hepatitis C and this should also be tested for at this stage.

A urine toxicology screen should be performed with the woman's consent, to confirm the drug history she has given and what the risks to the fetus may be.

❗ ILLEGAL DRUG USE RISKS

Crack cocaine: Crack cocaine use is associated with placental abruption and hence increased risk of perinatal death or prematurity. It is also known to cause intrauterine growth restriction by way of arterial vasoconstriction.

Heroin: Opiates are not teratogenic but are associated with intrauterine growth restriction and premature delivery.

Cannabis: Cannabis is not known to have specific risks in pregnancy, but the tobacco use associated and the possibility of other associated drug use makes it an important risk factor.

Tobacco: Tobacco use is associated with fetal growth restriction, low birth weight, abruption and stillbirth. There is also the risk of respiratory disease in the infant from passive smoking.

Management of the Pregnancy

Multidisciplinary Team

Most units have a specialist team for management of drug-using women in pregnancy. This should include specialists in substance misuse, a social worker, a specialist midwife and an interested obstetrician.

Opiate Replacement

The woman needs to be encouraged to engage more fully with the methadone replacement programme. This may well mean increasing the methadone regime to allow her to stop the street heroin. Once this has been achieved then she can gradually reduce the dose needed, with appropriate support. It is better to be still taking a maintenance dose of methadone through the pregnancy than to try and stop too quickly, resulting in unquantifiable amounts of illegal drugs being taken during the pregnancy.

Fetal Monitoring

The fetus should be assessed for growth during the pregnancy in view of the increased risk of intrauterine growth restriction.

Delivery

Labour should be managed as for any non-drug-using woman. The difference may be that the usual doses of opiates needed for analgesia (epidural or systemic) may be insufficient and need to be titrated up to ensure adequate pain control.

Fetal blood sampling should be avoided in labour due to the risk of vertical transmission of hepatitis B antigen.

Postpartum

The baby should be administered hepatitis B immunoglobulin at delivery and be given the accelerated hepatitis B immunization course.

Babies of opiate-using mothers may have initial respiratory depression as a result of the opiates but then develop withdrawal symptoms. They need immediate transfer to the neonatal unit for management of the symptoms, with reducing doses of opiates.

Issues of care for the baby should be established between the social services, medical team and the parents, prior to delivery.

 KEY POINTS

- Women who use illegal drugs have high-risk pregnancies.
- A team approach that encourages trust and engagement from the woman is likely to be most effective.
- Fetal growth should be monitored and the fetus transferred to the neonatal unit at delivery for management of respiratory depression and opiate withdrawal.

CASE 51: ANTENATAL SCREENING

History

A woman aged 23 years is referred by her general practitioner to the antenatal clinic at 12 weeks in her first pregnancy. She has booked late having only just discovered she is pregnant. She separated from her partner of 2 years a few weeks ago but is supported by her family and friends. She has no significant medical history and is one of four siblings. On direct questioning her mother apparently had a stillbirth attributed to some form of congenital abnormality 28 years ago. Otherwise the pregnancy is assessed to be low risk.

She is offered a screening test for Down's syndrome, which she agrees to. This is performed at 12 weeks 2 days' gestation.

 INVESTIGATIONS

Combined test for Down's syndrome:

- Pregnancy-associated plasma protein-A (PAPP-A): 0.4 multiples of the mean (MoM).
- Free beta-human chorionic gonadotropin (β-hCG): 1.7 multiples of the mean (MoM).
- Nuchal translucency: 2.9 mm.

Overall Down's syndrome risk calculated as 1 in 118.

? **QUESTIONS**

- What tests are available for screening for Down's syndrome and how accurate are they?
- How would you counsel this woman about her options now?

DOI: 10.1201/9781003386933-55

ANSWER 51

Screening for Down's Syndrome

PAPP-A, free β-hCG and ultrasound nuchal translucency thickness (NT) are used in combination as the 'combined' test, one of the screening tests available to detect Down's syndrome. Down's syndrome is associated with a decreased level of PAPP-A and increased level of NT and free β-hCG.

Serum marker levels are however affected by other variables. For example PAPP-A is decreased in heavier women, about 60 per cent higher in Afro-Caribbean and about 20 per cent lower in women who smoke, though these factors are taken account of in the risk assessment.

Other screening tests include the 'triple test', 'quadruple test' and 'integrated test'. All such tests aim for a detection rate of at least 90 per cent of affected fetuses and a screen positive rate of less than 2 per cent of the unaffected fetuses.

The assessment of 'high' or 'low' risk is dependent on the viewpoint of the individual, but risk higher than 1 in 150 is generally considered 'high risk'. Such women should be offered a diagnostic test.

Counselling

The woman should be counselled through the following options.

Expectant Management

- The woman may choose not to have any further testing and accept the chance of a baby with Down's syndrome.
- Detailed ultrasound scan: At 20 weeks, features of Down's syndrome (skull abnormalities, ventriculomegaly, atrial septal defect, duodenal atresia, echogenic bowel, hydronephrosis and short limbs) may be apparent on detailed anomaly scan. If none of these 'soft markers' are found then the woman might choose still to avoid further diagnostic tests.

Diagnostic Tests

- *Chorionic villous sampling (CVS)*:
  - Performed 11 to 14 weeks' gestation
  - Ultrasound guidance
  - Sample of placental tissue collected generally using needle inserted through the abdominal wall
  - Small risk of miscarriage (about 1 per cent) associated with the procedure
  - Inconclusive result in 1 per cent of cases (so amniocentesis then required)
- *Amniocentesis*:
  - Performed any time from 15 to 16 weeks' gestation
  - Ultrasound guidance
  - Sample of amniotic fluid collected using needle inserted through the abdominal wall
  - Small risk of miscarriage (about 1 per cent)
- *'Nonnonvasive prenatal testing (NIPT)'*: This more recently developed test detects cell-free fetal DNA in a sample of maternal blood from 10 weeks' gestation. It is used to identify

the common trisomies (21, 18, 13) and fetal gender. This is useful as a negative test means no further testing is required. However, if a positive result occurs then invasive testing is recommended to confirm the diagnosis.

Women's decisions depend on many factors. Some will want to know the diagnosis in order to consider termination of pregnancy, whereas other couples may not opt for termination but wish to be prepared for a baby with Down's syndrome (and any medical needs it may have, such as cardiac abnormalities) without the ongoing uncertainty throughout the duration of the pregnancy. Time for discussion and sensitivity to the woman's own situation are imperative in counselling.

KEY POINTS

- The possibility of screening for Down's syndrome should be considered with all women regardless of age.
- Women who choose not to undergo screening or diagnostic tests should have this choice respected.
- Screening tests produce a risk for an individual pregnancy being affected by a chromosomal abnormality, following which a woman may choose to undergo a diagnostic test.
- Diagnostic tests are chorionic villus sampling and amniocentesis.

CASE 52: EPILEPSY IN PREGNANCY

History

A 24-year-old woman attends for prepregnancy counselling. Her general practitioner referral letter is shown.

Dear Doctor

Please could you see and advise this young woman who wishes to start a family in the near future?

She was diagnosed with grand mal epilepsy when she was 12 and has been on medication since then. She was initially under a paediatric neurologist but for the last 6 years has been under my care at the practice. Her current treatment regime includes sodium valproate, phenytoin and lamotrigine. She last had a fit around 1 month ago.

I would be grateful if you could see her to discuss the management of any pregnancy. She has never been pregnant before.

Yours sincerely,

? | **QUESTIONS**

- What specific risks are there in pregnancy for this woman?
- How should she be managed?

ANSWER 52

The incidence of epilepsy in women of child-bearing age is approximately 1 in 150. The risks of epilepsy in pregnancy can be divided into risks to the mother and to the fetus.

Risks to the Mother

Increased plasma volume causes reduced drug levels and a possible increase in fits. Other causes of increased fit frequency during pregnancy include excessive tiredness and hyperemesis. Some women also decide to stop their medication because of fears of adverse effects on the baby, although this may actually increase the risk to the baby as a result of a higher likelihood of prolonged fits. The most serious risk to a woman with epilepsy is of Sudden Unexplained Death from Epilepsy (SUDEP). The number of women dying from this has increased in recent years.

Risks to the Fetus

There is an increased risk of congenital abnormality due to antiepileptic drugs, and this is directly related to the number of medications, type of medication and the dose. Carbemazepine and lamotrigine are accepted as the safest medications with sodium valproate known to be the most teratogenic. There is also an intrinsic increased risk of epilepsy in the offspring of an epileptic mother, and during the pregnancy the fetus is also at risk of fetal hypoxia from uncontrolled maternal epilepsy.

Management Principles

Prepregnancy

- Refer for neurology opinion to optimise medication, aiming for the fewest medications necessary. Do not stop medication prior to neurological input.
- Advise the woman to continue her medication during pregnancy, as having an increased number of fits is likely to increase the risk of fetal hypoxia as well as the risk of harm to the woman herself.
- Prescribe preconceptual folic acid (5 mg daily rather than 400 mg) to minimize the risk of neural tube defects and prevent folate deficiency seen with anti-epileptic regimes.

Antenatal

- Plan for joint medical and obstetric care.
- A woman who has had seizures in the previous year is more at risk during the pregnancy and needs to be monitored more closely.
- Advise the woman to take showers instead of baths to minimize the risk of drowning if a fit occurs in the bath.
- In addition to a detailed anomaly scan arrange fetal echocardiography at around 18–20 weeks to assess for cardiac abnormalities associated with anti-epileptics.
- All babies born to mothers taking anti-epileptic medication should have 1 mg intramuscular vitamin K recommended at birth.
- Adequate analgesia and close monitoring during labour and delivery are recommended in women with epilepsy especially as pain can trigger seizures in some women.

Postnatal

- Anticonvulsant therapy is not a contraindication to breast-feeding.
- Decrease medication doses as maternal physiology returns to normal.
- Adequate social support is vital and plans need to be made in advance for safe care of the infant (due to the risk of fits in the mother).

KEY POINTS

- Prepregnancy fits should be well controlled, aiming for a single drug regime.
- Epileptic medication is associated with an increased risk of congenital abnormality but the risk to the mother and baby of stopping medication usually outweighs the risk of fetal abnormality.
- Drug compliance during pregnancy must be emphasized.

CASE 53: OBESITY IN PREGNANCY

History

A woman has been referred for a hospital antenatal appointment at 16 weeks' gestation. This is her first pregnancy. She is 38 years old.

She booked for antenatal care with the midwife at 7 weeks and the only significant risk factor identified was that her BMI was 36 kg/m². She has always been overweight and considers her current weight as about normal for her. There is no significant past medical or gynaecological history.

Examination

Weight is 95 kg. Blood pressure is 145/88 mmHg. The uterus is not palpable on abdominal palpation but hand-held Doppler ultrasound reveals a fetal heartbeat of 155/min.

 INVESTIGATIONS

Urinalysis: Negative

Booking bloods:

- Syphilis: Negative
- HIV: Negative
- Hepatitis B: Negative
- Rubella: Immune
- Random blood glucose: 4.7 mmol/L
- Blood group A: positive
- Haemoglobin 131 g/L

? **QUESTIONS**

- How will you advise this woman about the possible effects of obesity on her pregnancy?
- What specific management plans should be put in place for her in view of the BMI?

DOI: 10.1201/9781003386933-57

ANSWER 53

Obesity in pregnancy is defined as BMI of greater than 30 kg/m² at first antenatal appointment and occurs in up to 20 per cent of women. Twenty-seven per cent of maternal deaths occur in obese women, and most adverse maternal and fetal outcomes are overrepresented in obese women.

Advice on Effects of Obesity on Pregnancy

Obese women should be sensitively advised of the increased risk of the following disorders in pregnancy: gestational diabetes (two- to threefold), hypertensive disorders (two- to threefold), venous thromboembolism (ninefold), slow labour and caesarean section (twofold), postpartum haemorrhage (twofold) and wound infection (twofold).

Fetal risks of maternal obesity include increased congenital abnormality (60 per cent increased risk), prematurity (20 per cent increased risk), macrosomia (two- to threefold), shoulder dystocia (threefold), stillbirth (twofold) and neonatal death (twofold).

Specific Pregnancy Management for This Woman

Preconception Advice

Ideally this woman should have had preconceptual information and advice regarding the pregnancy risks, with weight loss support offered prior to conception. She should have been prescribed folic acid at the higher dose of 5 mg daily at least 1 month before conception due to the higher incidence of neural tube defects in babies of obese mothers. Similarly, as an obese woman she is more likely to be vitamin D deficient and should have vitamin D supplementation during pregnancy and breast-feeding although how this affects outcomes remains uncertain.

Management in Pregnancy

- Anaesthetic consultation should be arranged to discuss the possible increased difficulty with venous access, regional anaesthesia or general anaesthetic.
- Antenatal thromboprophylaxis should be considered taking into consideration other risk factors for VTE.
- Increased frequency of antenatal blood pressure measurements should be arranged and a large cuff used if necessary for accurate assessment.
- Gestational diabetes screen (glucose tolerance test) should be performed by 28 weeks.
- With regard to planning for delivery, this woman should be advised to have a hospital birth (not home birth) due to increased maternal and fetal risks.
- Although a caesarean is more likely than in a non-obese woman, in view of the increased risks associated with operative delivery, a vaginal birth should be encouraged. Obesity is however an independent risk factor for shoulder dystocia and this should be discussed antenatally.
- Early intravenous access should be established in labour and there should be active management of the third stage, due to postpartum haemorrhage risk.
- Throughout the pregnancy she should be given advice on healthy diet and encouraged to lose weight between pregnancies.

CASE 54: GLUCOSE TOLERANCE TEST

History

A woman attends the antenatal day assessment unit to discuss the result of her glucose tolerance test. She is 42 years old and this is her sixth pregnancy. She has previously had three caesarean sections, one early miscarriage and a termination of pregnancy. All booking tests were normal as were her 11–14-week and anomaly ultrasound scans.

The woman is of Indian ethnic origin but was born and has always lived in the UK. She is now 26 weeks' gestation and her midwife arranged an oral glucose tolerance test because of a family history of type 2 diabetes (her father and paternal aunt).

Examination

The BMI is 31 kg/m². Blood pressure is 146/87 mmHg. The symphysiofundal height is 29 cm and the fetal heart rate is normal on auscultation.

 INVESTIGATIONS

Urinalysis: Glycosuria ++

Glucose tolerance test (75 g glucose drink):
- Pretest fasting blood glucose: 6.4 mmol/L
- 2 h blood glucose following glucose load: 11.3 mmol/L

? **QUESTIONS**

- What is the diagnosis and on what criteria can this be made?
- What are the principles of management for this patient?

ANSWER 54

The diagnosis is of gestational diabetes mellitus (GDM) and is based on the 2 h glucose concentration exceeding 7.8 mmol/L (World Health Organization [WHO] criteria). In this case, the diagnosis may also be made on the fasting blood glucose alone as this exceeds 5.6 mmol/L. Transient glycosuria is common in pregnancy and may occur after a glucose-rich drink or snack. Therefore the urinalysis alone is unhelpful in the assessment of this woman.

GDM occurs in up to 3 per cent of pregnant women depending on the ethnic diversity of the specific population. In some cases it may be the first presentation of previously undiagnosed diabetes.

! **RISK FACTORS FOR GDM**

- *Pre-existing*:
  - Obesity
  - Previous GDM
  - Family history of diabetes
  - Women with previously large babies or stillbirth
  - Increasing maternal age

! **ACQUIRED INDICATIONS FOR FORMAL GDM TESTING DURING PREGNANCY**

- *Occurring in this pregnancy*:
  - Glycosuria
  - Large for dates baby
  - Polyhydramnios

The importance of the diagnosis relates to both mother and fetus.

- *Effects on the fetus*:
  - Fetal macrosomia
  - Polyhydramnios
  - Neonatal hypoglycaemia
  - Neonatal respiratory distress syndrome
  - Increased stillbirth rate
- *Effects on the mother*:
  - Increased risk of traumatic delivery (e.g. shoulder dystocia)
  - Increased caesarean section risk
  - Increased risk of developing GDM in subsequent pregnancies
  - Fifty per cent increased risk of developing type 2 diabetes within 15 years

Management Principles

- Optimal control of maternal blood glucose minimizes the chance of fetal complications. Achieving this requires the multidisciplinary input of a diabetologist, specialist diabetes nurse, dietitian, specialist midwife and obstetrician.
- Dietary advice and counselling are the initial interventions (reduced fat and carbohydrate intake with weight control).

- Blood glucose monitoring at home should be initiated with pre- and postprandial levels at each meal.
- Oral hypoglycaemics (metformin) may be used prior to commencing insulin in women where diet control is not effective.
- If blood glucose measurements are repeatedly high, insulin should be commenced.
- The fetus should be monitored with regular ultrasound scans for growth and liquor volume (polyhydramnios being a sign of fetal polyuria secondary to excessive glucose level).
- Timing of delivery depends on blood sugar control, fetal size and medication being used to manage the diabetes. Women should be offered induction before 41 weeks' gestation (or 37–39 weeks if pre-existing type 1 or type 2 diabetes) and if this is declined a discussion with a senior member of the team about mode of delivery should be carried out.
- Sliding-scale insulin should be initiated in labour for women on insulin or whose blood sugar increases above certain thresholds.
- The insulin can be stopped immediately postpartum as normal glucose homeostasis returns rapidly after delivery in GDM.
- The fetus should be carefully monitored for neonatal hypoglycaemia.
- The mother should have a repeat glucose tolerance test 6 weeks postpartum to rule out pre-existing diabetes and yearly going forward due to increased risk of developing type 2 diabetes in the future.

 KEY POINTS

- Women should be informed that good blood glucose control throughout pregnancy reduces the risk of fetal macrosomia, trauma during birth (for her and her baby), induction of labour and/or caesarean section, neonatal hypoglycaemia and perinatal death.
- Gestational diabetes should initially be treated with dietary and weight advice. Insulin may be needed if blood glucose levels remain high.
- One-third of women with impaired glucose tolerance in pregnancy will go on to develop diabetes mellitus in the next 25 years.

CASE 55: ANTENATAL CARE

History

A woman attends a routine antenatal appointment at 31 weeks' gestation. She is 26 years old and this is her fourth pregnancy. She has three children, all spontaneous vaginal deliveries at term. Her third child is 18 months old and the delivery was complicated by a postpartum haemorrhage (PPH) requiring a 4-unit blood transfusion. This pregnancy has been uncomplicated to date, with normal booking blood tests, normal 11–14-week ultrasound and normal anomaly ultrasound scan.

She feels generally tired and attributes this to caring for her three young children. She reports good fetal movements (more than 10 per day).

Examination

Blood pressure is 126/73 mmHg.

 INVESTIGATIONS (BLOOD TESTS TAKEN AT 28 WEEKS)

		Normal Range for Pregnancy
Haemoglobin	78 g/L	110–140 g/L
Mean cell volume	68 fL	74.4–95.6 fL
White cell count	11.2×10^9/L	6–16×10^9/L
Platelets	237×10^9/L	150–400×10^9/L

Urinalysis: Negative
Blood group: A negative

No atypical antibodies detected.

? QUESTIONS

- What is the likely diagnosis and what are the implications for the pregnancy?
- What further investigations would you wish to arrange?
- How will you manage this woman for the last trimester of pregnancy?

DOI: 10.1201/9781003386933-59

ANSWER 55

The haemoglobin is significantly low even for pregnancy, and is associated with a low mean cell volume. This is usually due to iron-deficiency anaemia. Iron-deficiency anaemia usually occurs when the woman enters pregnancy with depleted iron stores, although she may not at that stage have low haemoglobin or any signs or symptoms suggestive of anaemia.

> **! IMPLICATIONS OF ANAEMIA IN PREGNANCY**
>
> - *Baby (possible)*:
>   - Low birth weight
>   - Neonatal anaemia
>   - Cognitive impairment
> - *Mother*:
>   - Antenatal
>   - Fatigue
>   - Fainting
>   - Dizziness
>   - Peripartum
>   - Increased risk of haemodynamic compromise
>   - Increased risk of postpartum haemorrhage
>   - Increased likelihood of transfusion

At delivery, blood loss is inevitable. This woman has additional risk factors of having her fourth delivery and having a history of PPH. As she is already very anaemic, she may decompensate easily if blood loss occurs, increasing her likelihood of hypovolaemic shock and need for emergency blood transfusion.

Further Investigation

Although the likely cause of these indices is iron deficiency, differential diagnoses include a mixed folate and iron deficiency, thalassaemia, chronic bleeding or anaemia of chronic disease (e.g. renal disease). A full history should therefore be taken to exclude chronic diseases and to elicit any family history of thalassaemia.

Iron deficiency should be demonstrated with findings of low mean cell haemoglobin (MCH) and low serum ferritin. Ferritin below 12 mg/L confirms the diagnosis. Serum and red cell folate should also be checked and the woman should be screened for haemoglobinopathies.

If chronic disease is suspected, then further investigations may be indicated such as renal and liver function tests for chronic disease, or gastrointestinal tract endoscopy for causes of chronic bleeding.

Further Management

Correction of Anaemia

- The woman should be prescribed ferrous sulphate 200 mg every other day. If iron tablets are not tolerated then alternatives include iron suspension or parenteral (intramuscular) iron injections. Parenteral iron can be associated with anaphylactic reactions but is generally well tolerated and a good alternative to blood transfusion.
- In cases where it is not possible to increase the haemoglobin level by iron supplementation, blood transfusion should be considered.
- An iron-rich diet should be encouraged.

Delivery

- At delivery, the woman should be considered at high risk of PPH and have an intra-venous cannula inserted in labour, with full blood count and group and save or cross-match available (depending on the haemoglobin level at that time).
- Active management of the third stage is essential (syntometrine, controlled cord traction) and an oxytocin infusion considered if bleeding is excessive or the uterus is suspected to be atonic.
- Following delivery, the woman should continue iron supplementation until iron stores (as assessed by ferritin level) are restored, even if haemoglobin is normal.

 KEY POINTS

- Anaemia (not physiological) must be investigated in pregnancy.
- If untreated, anaemia will worsen during pregnancy and blood loss at delivery may be catastrophic.
- Women with previous PPH must have active management of the third stage.

CASE 56: PREVIOUS CAESAREAN SECTION

History

A woman is referred to the obstetric antenatal clinic by the community midwife after the booking appointment revealed that she had had a previous emergency caesarean. You are the foundation year 2 doctor seeing her and you elicit the history and examine her.

She is 25 years old and pregnant with her second child. Her daughter was born 3 years ago by emergency caesarean section for failure to progress in labour due to an occipitoposterior position. The pregnancy had been uncomplicated and she had gone into spontaneous labour at 40 weeks 5 days. She had contractions for 24 h, and during this time she underwent artificial rupture of membranes and was given a syntocinon infusion for 8 h. The cervix dilated to 8 cm but she did not progress further despite regular strong contractions.

Following the emergency caesarean the baby was well, but the woman was readmitted to hospital after 7 days because of an infected wound haematoma for which she required intravenous antibiotics. The antibiotics altered the taste of the breast milk such that the baby refused to continue to feed from the breast and so subsequently had to have formula milk.

She now feels anxious that she might have to go through the same experiences again and is wondering whether she can request an elective caesarean section to avoid having another long labour and emergency procedure, with its associated complications.

She has had no other pregnancies and is generally fit and healthy. She is currently 16 weeks' gestation and has had a normal nuchal scan. Booking blood tests are normal.

Examination

The abdomen is distended, compatible with pregnancy. The low transverse scar is visible and is non-tender. The uterus is palpable to midway between the symphysis pubis and the umbilicus. The fetal heartbeat is heard with a hand-held Doppler machine.

> **?** | **QUESTION**
> - How should you advise and manage her?

DOI: 10.1201/9781003386933-60

ANSWER 56

The current average caesarean section rate in the UK is around 25 per cent. This means that many women are returning in subsequent pregnancies having had a previous caesarean section. In this case the woman has an otherwise low-risk pregnancy and the only factor to be considered at this stage is the planned mode of delivery.

She should be able to make an informed choice after appropriate information regarding vaginal birth after caesarean section versus planned caesarean section.

The important points for this woman to understand and to consider are summarized:

- *Vaginal birth after caesarean (VBAC)*:
  - Successful in up to 70 per cent of cases.
  - Emergency caesarean section rate is approximately 30 per cent.
  - One in 200 risk of uterine rupture (scar dehiscence) which increases to 1 in 100 with use of syntocinon.
  - Close cardiotocograph monitoring is needed, with intravenous access and full blood count and group and save serum available.
  - Induction of labour may be appropriate in selected women with previous caesarean section using mechanical methods such as balloon catheter cervical dilatation.
- *Planned caesarean section*:
  - Operative delivery is associated with higher risks of haemorrhage, infection, visceral damage and thrombosis.
  - The risk in every subsequent pregnancy is raised for conditions such as placenta praevia (low lying placenta) or placenta accreta (placenta that has invaded through the myometrium and is abnormally adherent).
  - Mobility and ability to care for child and baby are more impaired by caesarean section than vaginal delivery as average recovery time is 6 weeks.
  - Planned caesarean does avoid the possibility of an emergency procedure.
  - After two caesarean sections a further caesarean would be the recommended option if she has any more pregnancies.

The woman should be offered a further appointment towards the end of the third trimester to confirm her decision regarding mode of delivery and to check for any complications that might contraindicate vaginal delivery such as breech presentation, a large baby, scar tenderness or pre-eclampsia. One of the most important points in the consultation is to listen to her concerns about the previous delivery and what her fears might be. An empathetic approach will help her to feel confident about any decision she makes this time. It is also important to remember that the point of this consultation is not to convince the woman to deliver one way or another but to enable her to make an informed choice.

🔑 **KEY POINTS**

- Although low, the maternal morbidity and mortality are higher for caesarean section than for vaginal delivery.
- The chances of a successful vaginal delivery after a previous caesarean section are up to 70 per cent.
- A woman's experiences of previous deliveries are very important in counselling for any subsequent pregnancy and delivery.

CASE 57: GROUP B STREPTOCOCCUS

History

You are asked to see a woman in the antenatal assessment unit. She is gravida 4 para 1, having had a normal vaginal delivery 3 years ago, a first-trimester miscarriage and two first-trimester terminations.

She is currently 26 weeks' gestation. One week ago she was seen because she experienced vaginal bleeding. At the time a small cervical ectropion had been noticed and as the bleed had occurred postcoitally, it was assumed likely to be secondary to the ectropion.

However, according to protocol, she had vaginal and endocervical swabs sent and a full blood count and group and save sample requested.

🔍 INVESTIGATIONS

		Normal Range for Pregnancy
Haemoglobin	101 g/L	110–140 g/L
Mean cell volume	76 fL	74.4–95.6 fL
White cell count	8.0×10^9/L	$6–16 \times 10^9$/L
Platelets	183×10^9/L	$150–400 \times 10^9$/L

Blood group: A positive
No atypical antibodies detected.

Endocervical swab: Chlamydia negative; gonorrhoea negative
High vaginal swab: Candida – small numbers identified
Group B streptococcus: Positive culture

❓ QUESTIONS

- How would you interpret these results?
- How would you manage the pregnancy and delivery in light of these results?

DOI: 10.1201/9781003386933-61

ANSWER 57

The key results are:

- Mild anaemia
- Group B streptococcus carrier
- Candida

The anaemia is mild for pregnancy and as the mean cell volume is low, suggesting iron deficiency, it may be treated with ferrous sulphate 200 mg every other day, with repeat haemoglobin after 4 weeks. She should also be advised about an appropriate iron-rich diet (e.g. meat, lentils, spinach).

Candida organisms are present very commonly in the vagina, particularly in pregnancy. This should be treated (with vaginal clotrimazole) only if the woman is symptomatic (itching or lumpy discharge).

Group B Streptococcus (GBS)

GBS (*Streptococcus agalactiae*) colonization occurs in 25 per cent of women at some stage during their pregnancy. It is most likely to be an incidental finding. This is the most important result as there is a risk of GBS to the baby with an incidence of 1 in 2000 neonates being infected, with 6 per cent mortality.

> **! BABIES AT PARTICULAR RISK OF GBS INFECTION**
>
> - Previous baby affected by GBS
> - GBS in the vagina or urine at any stage during the current pregnancy
> - Preterm delivery
> - Prolonged rupture of membranes
> - Pyrexia in labour

In the UK, universal screening for GBS has not been shown to be effective in reducing neonatal death.

Management

Antenatal treatment does not seem to reduce the neonatal risk unless found in the urine (perhaps because of recolonization). However measures are taken to reduce transmission to the baby *at the time of delivery*:

- Intravenous benzylpenicillin (or clindamycin if allergic) should always be offered to the mother 4-hourly throughout labour.
- Neonatal care depends on the clinical scenario but if a well term baby is born to a mother who has received adequate intravenous antibiotics, then all that is required is observation of the baby for 12 hours postnatally.

> **🔑 KEY POINTS**
>
> - Candida infection is common in pregnancy and should be treated only if the mother is symptomatic.
> - GBS is the most common cause of serious bacterial infection in UK infants, with a mortality of around 6 per cent.
> - Antenatal treatment is generally not effective at reducing neonatal risk (unless GBS in the urine) but treatment at the time of delivery reduces perinatal morbidity and mortality.

CASE 58: TWIN PREGNANCY

History

A 37-year-old woman attends the antenatal clinic at 18 weeks' gestation. She is gravida 2 para 1, having had a spontaneous vaginal delivery at term 8 years ago. This current pregnancy was achieved through *in vitro* fertilization after four attempts (cycles). Two embryos were implanted. The first-trimester scan confirmed a twin gestation and noted a lambda sign between the gestational sacs. The anomaly scan is due in 2 weeks.

So far the woman has been feeling nauseated and tired but well.

Examination

The blood pressure is 120/78 mmHg. The fundus is palpable 2 cm above the umbilicus. Two separate fetal hearts are heard on hand-held fetal Doppler, one 143/min, the other 130/min.

🔎 INVESTIGATIONS

		Normal Range for Pregnancy
Haemoglobin	98 g/L	110–140 g/L
Mean cell volume	71 fL	74.4–95.6 fL
White cell count	5.3×10^9/L	$6–16 \times 10^9$/L
Platelets	204×10^9/L	$100–400 \times 10^9$/L

Urinalysis: Negative
Haemoglobin electrophoresis: Sickle trait (AS)
Blood group: A positive
Rubella antibody: Immune
HIV1/2: Negative
Hepatitis B: Negative
Syphilis: Negative

Twelve-week transabdominal ultrasound scan report: Two viable fetuses present, measuring 82 and 80 mm.

? QUESTIONS

- How would you interpret the results?
- What can the parents be told about the zygosity of the pregnancy?
- How would you monitor and manage this pregnancy?

ANSWER 58

The ultrasound confirms a twin pregnancy with a lambda sign (projection of placental tissue between the dividing membranes). This is suggestive of a dichorionic pregnancy. The woman is anaemic with a low mean cell volume suggestive of iron-deficiency anaemia. The only other investigation of note is that the woman has sickle trait.

Zygosity

Although the pregnancy appears dichorionic diamniotic (DCDA), this does not inform us about zygosity. A monozygotic pregnancy may be DCDA if the embryo has split at an early stage. One-third of monozygotic pregnancies are DCDA, two-thirds monochorionic diamniotic and around 1 per cent are monochorionic monoamniotic. A single implanted embryo may even split in an IVF pregnancy. Confirmation of dizygosity is by genetic analysis, or by observing that the fetuses are of different genders.

Monitoring

Twin pregnancies are associated with increased maternal risks of hyperemesis, anaemia, pre-term labour, antepartum haemorrhage, pre-eclampsia, gestational diabetes, thrombosis and caesarean delivery. The fetuses are at risk of intrauterine growth restriction, prematurity, still-birth or neonatal death, congenital anomalies and operative delivery.

! MONITORING IN TWIN PREGNANCIES

- Regular full blood count
- Close blood pressure and urinalysis monitoring
- Fetal growth surveillance from 24 weeks
- Screening for gestational diabetes

Management

In addition to routine antenatal care this woman needs:

- Information regarding the increased maternal and fetal risks with twin pregnancy
- Regular hospital antenatal assessment from the late second trimester
- Ferrous sulphate and folic acid supplementation if anaemic
- Discussion of mode of delivery (depending on growth and presentation of twins at around 36 weeks)
- Hospital delivery by 37 weeks
- Introduction to multiple pregnancy support groups

The woman has sickle trait and her partner should also be tested. If he is also sickle trait positive then prenatal testing of the babies should be offered to determine whether they are homozygous and therefore going to be affected by sickle cell disease.

🔑 KEY POINTS

- Chorionicity and amnionicity can be determined with high accuracy by ultrasound in the first trimester but unless the fetuses are seen to be of different sexes, the zygosity of dichorionic diamniotic twins can only be confirmed with genetic testing.
- Multiple pregnancies are high risk for both mother and babies, and close monitoring is essential for the early detection of problems.
- A woman with sickle cell trait whose partner is also sickle cell trait positive should be offered prenatal diagnosis by chorionic villus sampling, amniocentesis or cordocentesis.

CASE 59: CHICKEN POX EXPOSURE IN PREGNANCY

A woman has telephoned the antenatal clinic for advice. She is 16 weeks' gestation in her second pregnancy. She took her son to a birthday party yesterday and has now been telephoned by the party host to say that one of the other children at the party has just developed a typical chicken pox rash.

She is worried about the effect of chicken pox on her pregnancy.

 QUESTIONS

- What, if any, further questions do you need to ask her?
- What investigations should be performed?
- How will you advise and manage the case depending on the investigation results?

DOI: 10.1201/9781003386933-63

ANSWER 59

Chicken pox (caused by varicella zoster virus) is a very common, highly contagious and generally self-limiting mild childhood illness, mostly spread by respiratory droplets. Ninety per cent of antenatal women will have been previously infected with chicken pox and immunity can be demonstrated by the presence of varicella zoster virus (VZV) IgG antibodies in the serum.

Questions to Be Asked

- Does the woman know whether she has had chicken pox before?
- What was the nature of her contact with the affected child?
- What was the duration of her contact with the affected child?

When asked she can't remember whether or not she had chicken pox as a child. It was an indoor party and she herself had stayed at the party with her son for about 30 minutes.

Investigations to Be Performed

In many cases, a blood sample will have been retained from the antenatal booking blood tests that can be tested for VZV immunoglobulin (IgG). Otherwise the woman should be asked to have blood taken urgently for VZV IgG (ideally taken at the general practitioner's practice so that she does not attend the antenatal clinic and potentially infect other non-immune pregnant women).

Advice and Management

If the serum varicella IgG is positive then immunity is confirmed and the woman can be reassured that neither she nor her fetus is at risk of infection.

Maternal Risks

If the IgG is negative then she is not immune and more than 15 minutes in the same room as the infected individual is sufficient to place her at risk of infection. She should be given varicella immunoglobulin VZIG as soon as possible (effective if given up to 10 days after contact). She should then be advised that she is still potentially infectious and to avoid any other pregnant women during the infectious period of 8–28 days after exposure.

The risk of maternal varicella to the mother is greater than in the mild childhood form of the illness. Pneumonia, encephalitis and hepatitis are the potential complications. Maternal death is reported in 1 per cent of affected pregnant women (five times higher than in non-pregnant women). If she is infected then the rash would be expected to appear within 1–3 weeks. She must be advised to seek medical attention at the outset of a rash developing and should be prescribed acyclovir orally at the start of any symptoms. She must be referred to hospital for supportive care and intravenous acyclovir if chest symptoms, neurological symptoms or a haemorrhagic rash occur.

Fetal Risks

The risk of miscarriage is not increased in women who develop chicken pox in the first trimester. However fetal varicella syndrome (skin scarring, limb hypoplasia and neurological abnormalities) may occur in 1 per cent of fetuses of women infected up to 28 weeks, as a result of herpes zoster reactivation after the initial infection. Specialist fetal medicine ultrasound 5 weeks after initial infection may detect the anatomical abnormalities. If infection occurs before 12 weeks' gestation the chance of varicella syndrome is much lower.

Maternal infection at term carries the risk of varicella of the newborn which is a severe infection with up to 30 per cent mortality if untreated. The risk is approximately 30 per cent in infants of mothers infected 1–4 weeks before delivery, with highest risk conferred if infection is within 7 days of delivery. If possible delivery should therefore be delayed until after recovery from maternal infection to allow transplacental transfer of maternal antibodies to the fetus. VZIG should be given to the susceptible neonate.

If the woman is non-immune but does not develop the infection then vaccination should be recommended after delivery.

 KEY POINTS

- Chicken pox in pregnancy is potentially much more severe than in non-pregnant adults, with maternal death reported in up to 1 per cent of affected women.
- VZV is spread by respiratory droplets with same room contact for more than 15 minutes considered to place a non-immune woman at high risk.
- VZIgG should be given as soon as possible after exposure.
- Fetal risks of maternal chicken pox infection are fetal varicella syndrome (if mother infected before 28 weeks) or varicella of the newborn (if mother infected 1–4 weeks before delivery).

CASE 60: BLEEDING IN PREGNANCY

History

You are asked to review a nulliparous woman who has presented with vaginal bleeding at 39 weeks 5 days' gestation. Booking blood pressure was 123/72 mmHg. Her last midwife visit was 10 days ago when blood pressure was 130/76 mmHg.

This evening she noticed a small 'gush' of blood and discovered a bright red stain in her underclothes. She denies actual abdominal pain but reports some intermittent lower abdominal discomfort. The baby has been moving normally during the day.

Examination

She is warm and well perfused. Her blood pressure is 158/87 mmHg and heart rate 84/min. The symphysiofundal height is 36 cm and the fetus is cephalic with 3/5 palpable abdominally. Moderate uterine tenderness is noted. The uterus is soft but during the palpation two moderate uterine tightenings are noted. On speculum examination the cervical os is closed and there is a moderate amount of vaginal blood.

🔎 INVESTIGATIONS

Urinalysis: Protein +; blood ++; leucocytes negative; nitrites negative

The cardiotocograph (CTG) is shown in Figure 60.1.

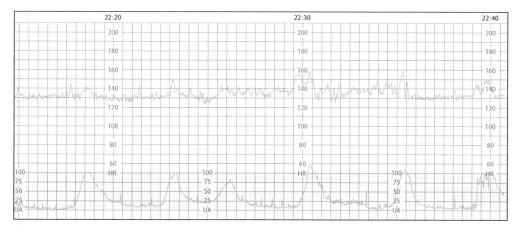

Figure 60.1 Cardiotocograph.

❓ QUESTIONS

- What is the diagnosis?
- How should this woman be managed?

DOI: 10.1201/9781003386933-64

ANSWER 60

The diagnosis is of placental abruption in view of the bleeding, uterine tenderness and irritability. The CTG is reassuring at present with baseline 130/min, normal variability, several accelerations and no decelerations. Regular frequent uterine activity is demonstrated on the tocograph.

!   COMMON CAUSES OF ANTEPARTUM HAEMORRHAGE (APH) AT TERM

- *Maternal blood*:
  - Blood-stained show
  - Bleeding placenta praevia
  - Placental abruption
  - Cervical ectropion
- *Fetal blood*:
  - Vasa praevia

A 'show' can be ruled out, as the blood is fresh rather than mucus-like and dark. Placenta praevia would have been detected at the anomaly scan, and bleeding placenta praevia is typically painless. She has no features suggesting infection, and vasa praevia bleeding would normally occur with rupture of membranes. Placental abruption is supported by the history of fresh bleeding and uterine irritability with the associated high blood pressure and proteinuria (pre-eclampsia is a cause of abruption).

Placental abruption may be major with catastrophic haemorrhage or, as in this case, be less dramatic. However caution should be maintained for two reasons: first, a small bleed may herald a larger bleed. Second, although some bleeding is revealed, there may be a more significant concealed bleed (with blood remaining within the uterine cavity rather than being visible). Pregnant women may not show any signs of hypovolaemic shock until a large amount of blood has been lost.

Management

Women with APH should always be admitted for observation. Initial management for this woman includes intravenous access, group and save, full blood count and clotting profile. Urea, electrolytes, urate and liver function tests should be sent, looking for abnormalities associated with pre-eclampsia. Blood pressure should be repeated at regular intervals and antihypertensives commenced if indicated.

Induction of labour may increase the chance of operative intervention, but the risk of expectant management in this case is that sudden and catastrophic further haemorrhage may occur. As the woman is over 37 weeks, there is little risk to the fetus of prematurity from induction and therefore immediate induction should be recommended. This woman has a high chance of needing an emergency caesarean section if she has any further bleeding or signs of fetal distress.

    KEY POINTS

- Placental abruption is a clinical diagnosis based on symptoms and examination.
- Blood loss caused by placental abruption may be concealed or revealed.
- A woman may not show signs of hypovolaemia until she has lost a large proportion of her blood volume.

CASE 61: BREECH PRESENTATION

History

You are asked to see a woman in the antenatal clinic. She is 37 years old and pregnant with her third child. Her previous children were both born by vaginal delivery after induction of labour for prolonged pregnancy.

First-trimester ultrasound confirmed her menstrual dates and she is now 37 weeks. At her last appointment at 36 weeks' gestation, the midwife suspected that the baby was in a breech presentation. An appointment has been made for an ultrasound assessment and to discuss the situation.

Examination

Blood pressure is 130/85 mmHg and abdominal examination suggests a breech presentation with the sacrum not engaged.

🔎 INVESTIGATIONS

Urinalysis: Negative

Ultrasound report:

- Indication for scan: Suspected breech presentation.
- Gestational age: 37 weeks 3 days.
- Extended breech presentation (hips flexed, knees straight).
- Estimated fetal weight: 3.2 kg.
- Placenta: High anterior.
- Liquor volume: Normal (amniotic fluid index 18 cm).

? QUESTIONS

- What are the options available to the woman?
- What management would you recommend in this case?

ANSWER 61

At 30 weeks the incidence of breech presentation is around 14 per cent, but is only 2–4 per cent by term.

> **! CAUSES AND ASSOCIATIONS FOR BREECH PRESENTATION**
>
> - Grand multiparity (lax uterus)
> - Uterine abnormality (bicornuate, septate, fibroids)
> - Placenta praevia
> - Polyhydramnios
> - Oligohydramnios
> - Multiple pregnancy
> - Congenital fetal abnormality
> - Prematurity

The three options available are:

1. Vaginal breech delivery
2. External cephalic version
3. Elective caesarean section

All three options should be discussed with the woman and her partner with important counselling points.

- *Vaginal breech delivery*:
    - Associated with an increased risk of hypoxic brain injury in singleton term fetuses than planned caesarean section, as demonstrated in the Term Breech Trial.
    - Carries a high chance of necessitating an emergency caesarean section.
    - Needs involvement of an experienced obstetrician with continuous fetal heart monitoring and ideally an epidural.
    - Should only be allowed if the labour progresses spontaneously – augmentation of breech labour is generally not recommended.
    - Contraindicated with placenta praevia, large baby, footling breech or a maternal condition such as pre-eclampsia.
- *External cephalic version*:
    - Involves using external manipulation of the fetus, encouraging the baby to turn to the cephalic presentation by way of pressure on the maternal abdomen.
    - Is often performed after giving a uterine relaxant such as terbutaline.
    - Carries a very small chance of abnormal fetal heart rate during or after the procedure which could necessitate an emergency caesarean section.
    - Has approximately 50 per cent success rate overall.
    - Some fetuses revert to breech position even after successful external cephalic version.
    - Contraindicated with previous caesarean section, other uterine surgery, pre-eclampsia, intrauterine growth restriction or oligohydramnios.
    - Can be painful.
- *Elective caesarean section*:
    - Is safer than vaginal breech delivery.
    - Is suitable where there are contraindications to external cephalic version.
    - Can be planned for in advance, which women may find more convenient.

- Does not necessarily mean a woman would need a caesarean section for any future pregnancy.
- Is associated with an overall higher maternal complication rate than vaginal delivery.

In this case, the woman should be recommended external cephalic version as soon as possible, with options for an elective caesarean section or possible trial of breech delivery if this is unsuccessful.

Postnatal paediatric review should have a focus on the baby's hips, with a neonatal ultrasound arranged within 6 weeks to rule out congenital hip dislocation (10–15 times more common in breech presentation).

KEY POINTS
- Breech presentation is associated with increased perinatal morbidity and mortality.
- If a woman has a frank breech at 37 weeks she should normally be offered external cephalic version, and if unsuccessful an elective caesarean section or possibly a vaginal breech delivery.

CASE 62: ANTENATAL SCREENING

History

A 31-year-old pregnant Bulgarian woman came to the UK 6 weeks ago with her English husband. As a result she booked late with the midwife at 31 weeks' gestation. This is her first ongoing pregnancy, having had two uncomplicated surgical terminations approximately 10 years ago. She reports a history of genital herpes diagnosed by her general practitioner several weeks ago. There is no relevant previous general medical history or family history.

She had an apparently normal first-trimester scan in Bulgaria before arriving in the UK and has had a normal anomaly scan in this hospital at 30 weeks' gestation.

Examination

Blood pressure is normal and symphysiofundal height is consistent with menstrual dates.

🔍 INVESTIGATIONS

		Normal Range for Pregnancy
Haemoglobin	117 g/L	110–140 g/L
Mean cell volume	87 fL	74.4–95.6 fL
White cell count	10.4 × 10⁹/L	6–16 × 10⁹/L
Platelets	389 × 10⁹/L	150–400 × 10⁹/L

Blood group: AB positive
Hepatitis B antigen: Negative
Rubella antibody: Immune
HIV1/2: Negative
T. pallidum enzyme immunoassay (EIA): Positive

❓ QUESTIONS

- What is the diagnosis?
- How should the woman be further investigated and treated?

ANSWER 62

Screening for syphilis is recommended for all pregnant women and *T. pallidum* EIA is a specific test for syphilis infection. The prevalence of infection is up to 0.3/1000 pregnant women in the UK. EIA tests that detect immunoglobulin G (IgG) or IgG and IgM, *T. pallidum* haemagglutination test and the fluorescent treponemal antibody-absorbed test (FTA-abs) are used generally for screening in pregnancy, as they are 98 per cent sensitive and over 99 per cent specific.

In cases with a positive screening test a second treponemal-specific confirmatory test should be sent to confirm the diagnosis. Caution is needed as treponemal-specific tests cannot differentiate syphilis from other treponemal disease (yaws, pinta and bejel).

The diagnosis in this woman is syphilis infection. She should be referred to a genitourinary medicine clinic for urgent assessment and treatment. She may have a genital ulcer (possibly misdiagnosed as herpes simplex) or features of secondary syphilis, but many women diagnosed are asymptomatic (latent syphilis).

Management
Treatment is with intramuscular penicillin daily for 10 days (doxycycline or erythromycin if penicillin allergic). Follow-up with a quantitative test (such as venereal disease research laboratory [VDRL]) should be used to confirm effective treatment and to monitor for reinfection. The woman's partner should be referred to the genitourinary medicine clinic for testing (45–60 per cent of partners will be infected).

The paediatricians should be informed at delivery to assess for signs of early congenital syphilis (usually developing in the first few weeks of life) and to arrange serological testing.

Untreated, 70–100 per cent of babies of mothers with syphilis infection will develop congenital syphilis, with a 30 per cent stillbirth rate.

!   **FEATURES OF CONGENITAL SYPHILIS**

- *Early congenital syphilis due to transplacental transfer of organisms (under 2 years):*
  - Condylomata lata rash
  - Snuffles
  - Lymphadenopathy
  - Hepatosplenomegaly
  - Ocular, renal and haematological involvement
- *Late congenital syphilis due to early structural damage (over 2 years):*
  - Interstitial keratitis
  - Hutchinson's incisors
  - Clutton's joints
  - Saddle nose deformity
  - Frontal bossing
  - Deafness

   KEY POINTS

- *T. pallidum* EIA is an enzyme immunoassay for syphilis.
- If untreated, pregnant women with syphilis will have a 30 per cent chance of a stillbirth and 70–100 per cent chance that the baby will have been infected with syphilis.

CASE 63: ELECTIVE CAESAREAN SECTION REQUEST

History

A 39-year-old woman has an appointment with you in the antenatal clinic to discuss the mode of delivery of her baby. She requests a caesarean section.

This is her first ongoing pregnancy, having had two first-trimester miscarriages in the last 3 years. She and her partner then tried for 12 months to conceive this pregnancy. The pregnancy however has been uncomplicated, with normal first trimester and anomaly scans and no medical concerns. She is now 34 weeks' gestation.

When asked why she wanted a caesarean section she says that she does not want to take any risks with this baby as she had been through the two miscarriages following which it has been so difficult to conceive this time. Her sister needed an emergency caesarean section a few months ago and recovered without complication.

The blood pressure is normal, there is no proteinuria and the symphysiofundal height is appropriate for the gestational age.

?	QUESTIONS

- How might you proceed in this consultation?
- What advantages and disadvantages will you put to this woman regarding her request for elective caesarean section for maternal request?
- Is it appropriate to agree to the woman's request for caesarean section without medical grounds?

DOI: 10.1201/9781003386933-67

ANSWER 63

In this consultation it is most important to understand what factors have brought this woman to make a request for caesarean section. For example as well as her concerns for the wellbeing of the baby, she may have a fear of labour ('tocophobia'), she may have feelings of not wanting to be out of control or she may be afraid of pain. All of these situations should be explored because the correct solution if there is, for example, a fear of labour, may be to address any underlying problem rather than bypassing it by performing caesarean.

It is then important to ascertain what she already knows about caesarean section in terms of the nature of the operation, the recovery time, the possible complications and the effect on future modes of delivery or any future surgery she may need. The woman needs evidence-based information and support. This information should include what the procedure involves, associated risks and benefits, and implications for future pregnancies and future birth after caesarean. She should also be informed of the risks and benefits of vaginal delivery. In counselling her it is important to take into account her individual circumstances, concerns and priorities.

Potential Advantages of Caesarean Section Delivery
- Predictable timing of delivery (unless labour occurs prior to the planned date of caesarean)
- Avoidance of the need for an emergency caesarean, which has higher complication rates
- Avoidance of the possibility of birth trauma such as shoulder dystocia to the baby and reduction in the rate of neonatal encephalopathy (NE) and postnatal death
- Reduction in the chance of pelvic floor weakness (although this occurs in part due to pregnancy itself and therefore incontinence and prolapse are not completely avoided by caesarean section)
- Lower rate of immediate postpartum haemorrhage
- Lower rate of injury to the vagina and perineum

Potential Disadvantages of Caesarean Section Delivery
- Increased rate of admission of baby to neonatal care unit
- Greater pain following abdominal surgery
- Possibility of intraperitoneal trauma to bowel or bladder at surgery
- Increased risk of wound infection
- Possibility of thrombosis (although this is minimized by the use of heparin prophylaxis)
- Longer hospital admission
- Increased likelihood of needing caesarean section in a subsequent pregnancy
- Very small increase in chance of hysterectomy for postpartum haemorrhage or of cardiac arrest

Are There Medical Grounds to Agree with the Request for Caesarean Section in This Case?
As long as the patient has been given all of the information and the time to discuss concerns then a caesarean section should be arranged for her. She should be informed of the possibility of going into labour before her caesarean section date (about 10 per cent chance) and the options available to her at that point, which include the choice of a trial of a vaginal delivery.

KEY POINTS

- UK National Guidance suggests that women requesting elective caesarean section may have this request agreed to having been given all the appropriate information to make an informed choice.
- Both immediate and long-term consequences of caesarean section should be explained when considering non-medically indicated caesarean section.

CASE 64: POSTPARTUM CHEST PAIN

History

A 32-year-old Sri Lankan woman presents complaining of chest pain, neck tightness and short-ness of breath 3 weeks after delivery. The symptoms have come on gradually over the last 2 days and are now severe. The pain is described as heavy and stabbing and is constant, though worse when she lies down and tries to sleep. The pain is not pleuritic and she says it radiates up into her neck. She does not have a cough or haemoptysis. When asked to describe the neck tightness she demonstrates that it is all around the neck but especially anterior, and is related to the difficulty breathing. The breathing difficulty occurs predominantly when the woman is trying to sleep or is sleeping – it has woken her several times during the night. She is now terrified of going to sleep and is actively stopping herself from doing so as she is certain that she will die if she does.

Prior to this episode the woman has always been fit and well with no previous medical history reported. The pregnancy was uneventful and she was admitted in spontaneous labour at 40 weeks. Cervical dilatation was slow and contractions were therefore augmented with syntocinon. Once fully dilated she had pushed for 90 min and subsequently underwent ventouse delivery of a healthy female infant. There was some difficulty establishing breast-feeding and bonding with the baby and she was finally discharged home on day 4 following delivery. Since going home she has stopped breast-feeding but is finding it difficult to sleep even when the baby is sleeping.

The woman has lived in the UK for 18 months but her husband has been here for 6 years. Currently her mother is also staying with them to help with the baby. Both the woman and her mother speak very little English and the husband is interpreting.

Examination

The woman appears thin and quiet, with little eye contact. When talking about the baby her affect appears flat and she does not look at or touch the baby during the consultation. She is apyrexial with blood pressure of 108/62 mmHg and heart rate 90/min. No signs of anaemia, cyanosis or oedema are detected and chest and cardiac examinations are normal. The uterus is just palpable in the lower abdomen.

🔍 INVESTIGATIONS

		Normal Range for Pregnancy
Haemoglobin	108 g/L	110–140 g/L
Mean cell volume	78 fL	74.4–95.6 fL
White cell count	5.3×10^9/L	$6–16 \times 10^9$/L
Platelets	237×10^9/L	$150–400 \times 10^9$/L

Electrocardiogram (ECG): Sinus rhythm, no abnormalities.
Chest X-ray: Normal heart and lung fields.
Oxygen saturation: 100 per cent on air.

Arterial Blood Gas		
pO_2	16 kPa	12–14 kPa
pCO_2	3.8 kPa	5–6 kPa

❓ QUESTIONS

- What is the likely diagnosis?
- What further questions would you wish to ask and what are the principles of management?

DOI: 10.1201/9781003386933-68

ANSWER 64

The symptoms initially sound possibly cardiac or respiratory in origin. However the story does not fit with any specific disease and the examination and investigations are all normal. The absolute fear of sleeping is an important piece of information as is the observed affect.

This woman is suffering from early postnatal psychosis. This occurs in 1 in 500 women with onset in the first 6 weeks post-delivery. The commonest symptoms are delusions (e.g. the thought that she is going to die) and hallucinations.

The condition should be distinguished from the two other main psychological/psychiatric post-natal conditions.

- *Postpartum blues*:
  - Tearfulness
  - Fatigue
  - Anxiety over their own or the baby's health
  - Feelings of inability to cope

This is very common (probably affecting approximately half of mothers) usually after the third postnatal day, and resolves spontaneously over a few days.

- *Postpartum depression*:
  - Low mood
  - Crying
  - Anxiety over the baby's health
  - Feelings of guilt towards the baby
  - Panic attacks
  - Excessive tiredness
  - Poor appetite

This occurs in 10 per cent of women, any time up to 6 months following delivery. It should be treated seriously with a suicide risk assessment and antidepressant medication as well as social and practical support.

Further Questioning

A trained interpreter should be sought rather than the husband who is involved in this case and may find it difficult to translate or address sensitive issues.

The woman should be asked for any previous personal or family history of mental illness or psychiatric treatment. She should then be asked more probing questions. How is her mood and appetite? Does she feel depressed? Does she have fears of harming herself?

Her relationship and attitudes to the baby are important – how does she feel about the baby? Is she finding the baby easy? Does she feel that the baby is healthy? Does she have any negative thoughts towards the baby such that it is bad or evil? Does she feel she might harm the baby?

Suicide is now the commonest cause of indirect maternal death, and non-English-speaking immigrants are particularly at risk as well as those aged over 30 years, with previous psychotic history, poor social support or traumatic delivery. This woman has three such risk factors.

The diagnosis should always be considered when symptoms do not appear to be backed up by the examination or investigations. Sometimes delusional symptoms or hallucinations are not elicited because the doctor fails to take a thorough history.

Management

Disease progression can be acute and this woman needs immediate referral to a mother and baby psychiatric unit for assessment and treatment. Depending on her feelings of harm towards herself or others, this may need to be under the Mental Health Act. Antidepressants, antipsychotics and possibly sedation may be needed. The baby may be at risk from neglect or harm secondary to the psychosis, so close supervision and support are essential. Recovery is expected within 2 months but repeat pregnancy and non-pregnancy-related episodes are common.

 KEY POINTS

- Postpartum psychosis is generally diagnosed in the community after discharge from hospital after delivery.
- It is unlikely that a woman herself will recognise the symptoms, and the condition can escalate rapidly.
- The condition should be treated as a medical emergency.
- Women with postpartum psychosis must be admitted to a mother and baby psychiatric unit, if need be under the Mental Health Act.

CASE 65: ANTENATAL ULTRASOUND

History

A 31-year-old woman attends a routine antenatal appointment at 28 weeks' gestation. She is para 2 having had two previous term vaginal deliveries, with the same partner. Her children are aged 4 and 2 years and weighed 3.7 and 3.6 kg, respectively, at birth. She reports no antenatal concerns, there is no abdominal pain, no vaginal bleeding and good fetal movements are reported.

Initial antenatal booking blood tests were normal, as were the first-trimester nuchal screen and 20-week anomaly scans.

She is a non-smoker and has abstained from alcohol during the pregnancy.

Examination

The woman appears well with no signs of oedema. Her BMI is 24 kg/m². Blood pressure is 115/74 mmHg.

The symphysiofundal height is 24 cm. The fetus is felt to be a cephalic presentation. Auscultation with hand-held Doppler confirms the fetal heartbeat to be 150/min.

 INVESTIGATIONS

Urinalysis: Negative
Ultrasound: Biparietal diameter and femur length are on the 10th centile. Abdominal circumference and estimated fetal weight are below the fifth centile. The liquor volume is normal. Umbilical artery resistance index is within normal range.

? **QUESTIONS**

- What are the possible causes of the small fetal size and what further investigations would you propose?
- How would you manage this pregnancy from now?

DOI: 10.1201/9781003386933-69

ANSWER 65

Intrauterine growth restriction is defined as predicted birth weight less than 10th centile for gestational age. The most common cause is uteroplacental insufficiency, commonly part of the pre-eclampsia process. However, there are multiple alternative causes.

Causes of Small for Gestational Age Fetus		
Maternal		*Fetal*
Chronic hypertension	Maternal smoking	Congenital infection
Pre-eclampsia	Excess alcohol	Chromosomal anomaly
Placental insufficiency		
Diabetes	Malnutrition	Constitutionally small fetus
Chronic renal disease	Hypoxic lung disease	

In this case, there is no evidence of hypertension or pre-eclampsia and as she has not changed partner and it is only 2 years since her last birth, it would be unusual for the woman to develop pre-eclampsia in this pregnancy. She has no personal or family history of diabetes, renal or respiratory disease. It is therefore likely that the fetus is small due to fetal rather than maternal factors.

Further Investigation

The baby may be constitutionally small but in light of the previous two babies being of normal birth weight, this is less likely.

A TORCH serum screen should be performed to identify maternal viral infection that may be associated with fetal growth restriction. This includes toxoplasmosis, rubella (if non-immune at booking), cytomegalovirus and herpes simplex. Other infections that may be associated with growth restriction include Epstein–Barr virus, syphilis, hepatitis, parvovirus and HIV.

Discussion about testing for chromosomal abnormalities should be had which may require invasive testing with amniocentesis.

Management of the Pregnancy

The management depends on the investigation results. If the infection screen reveals a recent maternal infection then the management involves close fetal medicine surveillance to determine appropriate timing of delivery and neonatal treatment.

If no cause for the growth restriction is found then serial ultrasound scans should be performed. Reduced amniotic fluid volume followed by increased resistance in the umbilical arteries is associated with adverse perinatal outcome in a growth-restricted fetus and development of these features can be used to determine timing and mode of delivery. If the umbilical artery doppler remains normal then delivery should be offered at 37 weeks. Where preterm delivery is indicated before 34 weeks' gestation, maternal corticosteroid injections should be considered to reduce the incidence of respiratory distress syndrome in the neonate.

 KEY POINTS

- Intrauterine growth restriction is caused most commonly by uteroplacental insufficiency.
- Serial growth scans should be carried out if IUGR is suspected.
- Tests for infection or chromosomal anomaly may be indicated for IUGR pregnancies where no other obvious cause is apparent.

CASE 66: HIV IN PREGNANCY

History

A 36-year-old Nigerian woman who has lived in the UK for 8 years attends the antenatal clinic. She had a daughter by spontaneous vaginal delivery at term 17 years ago and a termination of pregnancy 9 years ago. She and her partner have now been trying to conceive for 4 years.

Her last menstrual period was 11 weeks ago. There is no significant gynaecological history and last smear test was normal 2 years ago.

The woman saw the midwife for a routine antenatal booking appointment a week ago and no relevant past medical history was reported. All routine booking blood tests were accepted.

INVESTIGATIONS

		Normal Range for Pregnancy
Haemoglobin	119 g/L	110–140 g/L
Mean cell volume	77 fL	74.4–95.6 fL
White count	4.1×10^9/L	$6–16 \times 10^9$/L
Platelets	129×10^9/L	$150–400 \times 10^9$/L

Blood group: AB positive
Hepatitis B surface antigen: Negative
Syphilis: Negative
HIV1/2: Positive
Rubella: Immune
CD4: 175/mm^3
Viral load: 10,000 copies/mL

QUESTIONS

- What is the diagnosis?
- What is the next stage in management?
- What are the important points in the management of the pregnancy in view of the diagnosis?

ANSWER 66

The diagnosis is human immunodeficiency virus (HIV) infection. HIV screening in pregnancy is recommended for all women in the UK and the latest reported incidence was approximately 0.4 per cent in inner London and less than 0.1 per cent for the rest of the UK. It is particularly prevalent in women from Africa (2.5 per cent compared with <0.5 per cent in UK-born women). The vast majority of paediatric HIV cases in the UK result from mother-to-child transmission.

Unlike in this case, around 90 per cent of women with HIV are aware of their diagnosis prior to pregnancy. In this woman the low CD4 count suggests the need to commence treatment, but there are no AIDS-defining illnesses in the history.

Immediate Management

The woman needs to be informed of the suspected diagnosis and a second different confirmatory diagnostic test performed. She needs urgent referral to the genitourinary medicine specialist for further screening for other STIs and investigation for any HIV complications. She will need to start *Pneumocystis carinii* prophylaxis in view of the low CD4 count. All women with HIV need antiretroviral treatment during pregnancy. This woman should be commenced on combination antiretroviral therapy (cART) in view of her high viral load. Psychological counselling in relation to the diagnosis and the implications for her, her partner and her offspring (the fetus and her 17-year-old daughter) is very important.

Management of the Pregnancy

Pregnancy does not adversely affect the HIV disease process. The important consideration is therefore the prevention of transmission from mother to child. Untreated, approximately 25 per cent of infants of mothers with HIV will become infected. With appropriate measures, this is reduced to less than 1 per cent:

- *All HIV-infected women*:
  - Avoidance of breast-feeding
  - Oral zidovudine or triple drug post-exposure prophylaxis to the neonate for 2–4 weeks postnatally (depending on maternal viral load and treatment)
- *Women with viral load >50 HIV RNA copies/mL at delivery or viral load unknown*:
  - Intravenous zidovudine to the mother prior to delivery (ideally for 4 h)
  - Elective caesarean section

Thus women with undetectable viral load at term may aim for a vaginal delivery (in the absence of obstetric complications) as this has been shown to have no effect on the chance of infant infection in such cases.

Confidentiality is of paramount importance for women diagnosed antenatally with HIV, and coding systems in the obstetric notes can be helpful in alerting other medical staff to the diagnosis.

 KEY POINTS

- The incidence of HIV in pregnancy remains significant.
- To decrease vertical transmission all HIV-positive women should avoid breast-feeding and the neonate should be given 2–4 weeks' oral antiviral treatment.
- Depending on the individual situation, elective caesarean section and/or predelivery intravenous zidovudine are indicated in women with detectable viral load.

CASE 67: ITCHING IN PREGNANCY

History

A 36-year-old woman is complaining of itching. She is currently 34 weeks' gestation in her first pregnancy. The itching started 2 weeks ago and she had been using emollient cream to try and relieve it. Initially it was mainly over her soles and palms, although it is now more generalized. She is not aware of having changed her washing powder or soap recently and no one else in her family has been affected.

She has not experienced any abdominal pain although she does have Braxton Hicks contractions. There is no vaginal discharge or bleeding. She reports good fetal movements.

Examination

She looks well. Her blood pressure is 118/76 mmHg and pulse 82/min.

No rash is visible on the face, trunk, limbs, hands or feet except for a few excoriation marks.

The symphysiofundal height is 34.5 cm and the uterus is soft and non-tender. The fetus is cephalic with 4/5 palpable abdominally.

🔍 INVESTIGATIONS

		Normal Range for Pregnancy
Haemoglobin	103 g/L	110–140 g/L
Mean cell volume	80 fL	74.4–95.6 fL
Platelets	198 × 10⁹/L	150–400 × 10⁹/L
Sodium	132 mmol/L	130–140 mmol/L
Potassium	3.3 mmol/L	3.3–4.1 mmol/L
Urea	2.9 mmol/L	2.4–4.3 mmol/L
Creatinine	68 mmol/L	34–82 mmol/L
Alanine transaminase	40 IU/L	6–32 IU/L
Alkaline phosphatase	120 IU/L	30–300 IU/L
Gamma glutamyl transaminase	12 IU/L	5–43 IU/L
Bilirubin	8 mmol/L	3–14 mmol/L
Bile acid	24 mmol/L	0–14 mmol/L

Urinalysis: Nil abnormal detected.

❓ QUESTIONS

- What is the diagnosis?
- How would you further investigate and manage this woman?
- How will this diagnosis affect the pregnancy?

DOI: 10.1201/9781003386933-71

ANSWER 67

The woman is suffering from obstetric cholestasis (OC). This is a pregnancy-specific condition in which intrahepatic reduction of bile excretion from the liver causes a buildup of serum bile acids. It usually develops in the third trimester. The presenting complaint is itching (without rash) – most typically on the palms of hands and soles of feet. In more severe cases the liver function or coagulation becomes deranged, and if this occurs then other diagnoses such as HELLP syndrome (haemolysis, elevated liver enzymes and low platelets – a severe form of pre-eclampsia) or hepatitis should be considered.

There is no long-term harm to the mother. The effect on the baby however is potentially much more serious with an association between OC and stillbirth.

Investigations

A viral hepatitis screen should be carried out to confirm no infective cause of the abnormal liver function.

Abdominal ultrasound should be performed to exclude gall stones or other causes of hepatic obstruction. Fetal ultrasound may be performed for maternal reassurance.

Management

Symptomatic relief is obtained from chlorpheniramine (antihistamine). Ursodeoxycholic acid can be given to relieve itching in more severe cases, as it reduces serum bile acids, however there is no evidence that it helps reduce the risk of stillbirth.

Discussion about timing of delivery should be had with the woman depending on the severity of symptoms and degree of abnormality in bloods but induction is recommended by 40 weeks at the latest.

Postnatal Advice

Maternal liver function returns to normal after delivery, but the mother should be warned that recurrence may occur in a subsequent pregnancy (50 per cent) or with use of the combined oral contraceptive pill.

 KEY POINTS

- Itching in pregnancy may be due to obstetric cholestasis.
- In severe cases maternal liver and coagulation function can become deranged, but usually the major risk is to the fetus.
- There is a high risk (50 per cent) of recurrence in future pregnancies.

CASE 68: TIREDNESS IN PREGNANCY

History

A 27-year-old woman attends the antenatal clinic at 19 weeks' gestation in her first ongoing pregnancy, having had a termination at age 22 years. She is now happy to be pregnant.

She booked with the midwife at 8 weeks and has had normal booking bloods, blood pressure and ultrasound scan.

She experienced nausea and vomiting until 14 weeks' gestation. This has now settled but she remains very tired and feels that she is gaining excessive weight in the pregnancy. She also feels cold for much of the time, which surprises her as she understood that pregnant women tend to feel hot.

Examination

The woman appears lethargic and of low mood. Her blood pressure is 115/68 mmHg and heart rate 58/min. Abdominal examination is unremarkable, with the fundus palpable at the umbilicus.

INVESTIGATIONS

		Normal Range for Pregnancy
Haemoglobin	102 g/L	110–140 g/L
Mean cell volume	78 fL	74.4–95.6 fL
White cell count	7.9 × 10⁹/L	6–16 × 10⁹/L
Platelets	272 × 10⁹/L	150–400 × 10⁹/L
Thyroid-stimulating hormone (TSH) antibody	15 mu/L	0.5–7 mu/L
Free thyroxine (T₄)	6 pmol/L	11–23 pmol/L

QUESTIONS

- What is the diagnosis and what features will you look for on examination?
- What are the implications for the mother and baby in pregnancy?
- How should the condition be managed?

DOI: 10.1201/9781003386933-72

ANSWER 68

The full blood count shows mild anaemia, with relatively low mean cell volume. This is not significant enough however to account for the symptoms described.

The thyroid function tests confirm the clinical diagnosis of hypothyroidism. There is no history of radioactive iodine or surgical treatment, and Hashimoto's thyroiditis is unlikely as there has been no history of a hyperthyroid episode. This case therefore probably represents idiopathic myxoedema.

The symptoms of tiredness, cold intolerance and weight gain may all relate to the hypothyroidism. In addition she should be asked specifically about dry skin, coarse hair, depression or constipation.

Examination may reveal relative bradycardia, blunted deep tendon reflexes or goitre.

Implications for the Pregnancy and Management

Hypothyroidism occurs in approximately 1 in 100 pregnancies, but this case is unusual in that the diagnosis is made in pregnancy.

Myxoedematous coma is a very rare consequence of hypothyroidism, associated with a high mortality rate. It is a medical emergency managed by supportive care and thyroxine supplementation. In the absence of a coma, thyroxine replacement is still needed and should be titrated to the TSH and T_4 results.

In pregnancy, the thyroxine requirement may increase, and the TSH and T_4 should be checked every trimester once a maintenance regime has been established. The aim should be to keep the TSH less than 5 mu/L.

(Although thyroid-binding globulin increases in pregnancy, there is a compensatory rise in triiodothyronine [T_3] and T_4 production such that the levels of free T_3 and free T_4 remain similar to non-pregnant values.)

The Fetus

Untreated hypothyroidism is associated with an increased risk of infertility, miscarriage, stillbirth and pre-eclampsia. The fetal and neonatal outcome is however generally good in women diagnosed and treated appropriately. Anti-TSH antibodies may very rarely cross the placenta and cause neonatal hypothyroidism, and this should be suspected if there are signs of neonatal goitre.

 KEY POINTS

- Untreated hypothyroidism is associated with infertility, miscarriage, low birth weight, fetal loss, pre-eclampsia and anaemia.
- Women established on thyroxine should have thyroid function monitored once in each trimester of pregnancy.

CASE 69: DIABETES IN PREGNANCY

History

A 20-year-old woman is pregnant for the first time. The pregnancy is unplanned and the partner has left but she is supported by her mother and has decided to continue.

She was diagnosed with type 1 diabetes at age 15 years. She has been taking long-acting and short-acting insulin under the care of her general practitioner (GP), but the referral letter suggests that she has not always been compliant.

She had a positive pregnancy test 2 weeks ago and her GP has referred her urgently to the antenatal clinic for review in view of the diabetes. By her dates she is now 7 weeks and 5 days' gestation. She has no other significant gynaecological or medical history.

Examination

The woman has a BMI of 29 kg/m². Blood pressure is 131/68 mmHg and pulse is 81/min.

🔍 INVESTIGATIONS

		Normal Range
Haemoglobin (Hb)A$_{1c}$	55	<45
Urinalysis: glucose ++		

❓ QUESTIONS

- What further investigations need to be arranged?
- Outline the principles of management of the pregnancy.

DOI: 10.1201/9781003386933-73

ANSWER 69

The investigations can be divided into those for maternal and for fetal wellbeing:

- *Maternal wellbeing*:
  - Baseline urea and electrolytes
  - Pre- and postprandial capillary blood glucose measurements
  - Retinal assessment if not performed in the last 12 months
- *Fetal wellbeing*:
  - Early pregnancy viability scan (increased risk of miscarriage in diabetic women)
  - Detailed anomaly ultrasound examination at 20 weeks
  - Fetal echocardiography (increased risk of all fetal abnormalities in diabetic offspring)
  - Regular third-trimester growth scans

Diabetic (type 1) pregnancies may be affected by an increase in a range of complications as well as fetal abnormalities. However, optimal control of blood sugar is thought to reduce the complication risk to near that of a non-diabetic pregnancy, so a large proportion of management is aimed at maintaining very tight blood glucose control. In this particular case, the history, HbA_{1c} and presence of glycosuria suggest that the woman has generally poor control until now, providing a particular challenge to management of this pregnancy.

! MANAGEMENT PRINCIPLES IN MATERNAL INSULIN-DEPENDENT DIABETES

- *Antenatal*:
  - Immediate change to an increased insulin-dosing regime using more frequent doses to adapt to the increasing demand in pregnancy.
  - Aim to keep fasting blood glucose between 3.5 and 5.9 mmol/L and 1 h postprandial blood glucose below 7.8 mmol/L throughout the pregnancy.
  - Advise women of the risk of hypoglycaemia and hypoglycaemia unawareness in pregnancy.
  - Multidisciplinary care with endocrinologist/diabetologist, dietitian, specialist diabetic nurse, obstetrician and midwife with special interest in diabetic pregnancies.
  - Full hospital care with regular review, usually every 2 weeks, or more frequently if control remains poor.
  - Increase in insulin requirements expected throughout the pregnancy.
  - Regular ultrasound assessment from 28 weeks for fetal growth and liquor volume, in view of the risk of macrosomia and polyhydramnios, secondary to fetal hyperinsulinaemia.
  - Consideration of induction of labour at 38 weeks to reduce the risk of sudden stillbirth.
- *In labour*:
  - Sliding-scale insulin regime in labour (or during caesarean section).
  - Aim for vaginal delivery unless contraindicated by obstetric factors.
- *Postnatal*:
  - Early blood glucose checks and feeding of the baby in view of its hyperinsulinaemic state.
  - Reduction of maternal insulin regime to the prepregnancy regime immediately after delivery.
  - If breast-feeding then insulin will need to be reduced further as this increases the risk of hypoglycaemia.

KEY POINTS

- Type 1 diabetes pregnancies are high risk for mother and fetus and need specialist diabetes and obstetric input. Very close blood glucose control, if achieved, should reduce the complication rate to near that of a non-diabetic mother.
- Fetal complications include miscarriage, congenital abnormality, macrosomia, still-birth and shoulder dystocia.

Section 5

PERIPARTUM CARE AND OBSTETRIC EMERGENCIES

CASE 70: PALPITATIONS AND SHORTNESS OF BREATH IN PREGNANCY

A 44-year-old woman presents to obstetric triage at 37 weeks' gestation in her first pregnancy reporting heart palpitations. She has never experienced these prior to pregnancy. The palpitations are worse when she is lying down at night but she has been noticing them increasingly throughout the past few days. She also reports getting more gradually short of breath over the last week and has been struggling to breathe when lying flat. At night she has been coughing.

Her shoes no longer fit her and she has had to take her wedding rings off in the last week for comfort.

This was an IVF pregnancy with a donor egg. Prior to pregnancy she was well with no underlying health conditions. She moved to the UK from Nigeria for work 2 years ago.

Examination

The woman appears short of breath at rest but is able to complete full sentences. Her observations are as follows: Heart rate 110/min, respiratory rate 20/min, blood pressure 120/80 mmHg, temp 36.0 degrees, SpO$_2$ 96 per cent on air.

Examination

HS: I + II + pansystolic flow murmur.

Chest: Reasonable air entry and lung fields clear apart from bibasal crepitations.

Abdomen: Soft and non-tender, distended appropriate to gestation.

Peripheries: Capillary refill time <2 seconds, pitting oedema to the thighs.

🔍 INVESTIGATIONS

ECG – Sinus tachycardia.
CXR – Bilateral pleural effusions seen.
Echo – Left ventricular ejection fraction 30 per cent, structurally normal.

❓ QUESTIONS

- What is the diagnosis?
- What is the management?
- What is the prognosis for this patient?

ANSWER 70

This is a classic presentation of peripartum cardiomyopathy, a condition unique to pregnancy. It usually presents in late pregnancy or peripartum. It is associated with extremes of age (old or young), underlying hypertension, increased parity, African ethnicity and obesity although it can also present in women with no risk factors. Orthopnoea, tachycardia and gross oedema are the classic presenting features and warrant swift investigation. These women may deteriorate quickly and input from a multidisciplinary obstetric, anaesthetic and cardiology team is vital.

In this case, the woman is in acute heart failure and management should be as such with beta-blockers, furosemide and discussion of angiotensin converting enzyme (ACE) inhibitors (if the benefit outweighs risk). Timing of delivery should be discussed and a postnatal management plan put in place with a very low threshold for transfer to a high dependency or intensive care unit for optimal care.

The outcome can be poor for this condition with a mortality rate from 1 to 30 per cent depending on patient population studied, so it is vital to have a high level of suspicion in any woman presenting with cardiac symptoms. Ongoing cardiac postnatal follow-up should be arranged for such women and very close MDT care is required if they conceive again.

 KEY POINTS

- Any woman presenting with orthopnoea, persistent tachycardia or gross oedema should be investigated for cardiomyopathy.
- Cardiomyopathy is associated with a high maternal mortality risk.
- Multidisciplinary care is vital in women with obstetric medical problems such as peripartum cardiomyopathy.

CASE 71: REDUCED FETAL MOVEMENTS

History

A 34-year-old in her first pregnancy presents to the obstetric triage at 32 weeks with a 6-hour history of reduced fetal movements. This is her first presentation with this symptom. She is generally well and has had midwifery care so far in this pregnancy. She reports that she normally feels her baby move more in the evenings but not so much during the day. She does not have any abdominal pain, vaginal bleeding or history of vaginal fluid leak.

Her last scan was the anomaly scan at 20 weeks and was normal. She had normal booking bloods and low-risk combined screening at 12 weeks. Her 28-week bloods were normal.

Her cardiotocography (CTG) is shown in Figure 71.1.

? QUESTIONS

- What would you recommend in this case?
- What would you do if she was 40 weeks' gestation at this point?

DOI: 10.1201/9781003386933-76

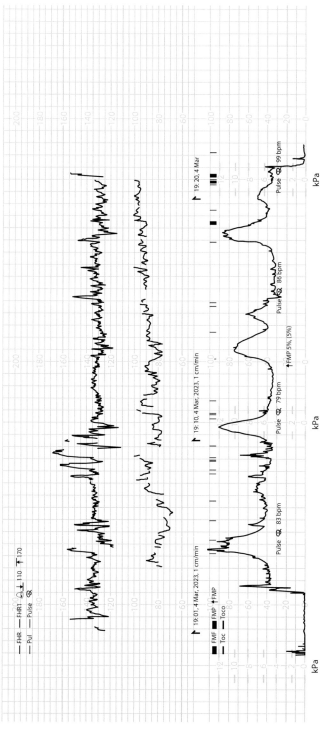

Figure 71.1 Normal CTG.

ANSWER 71

Management

Any woman who is concerned about reduced fetal movements should be invited into the maternity unit for assessment of fetal wellbeing. This is because reduced fetal movements is one of the only symptoms seen in women who later go on to have a stillbirth, so it is vital that any concerns about movements are taken seriously. An initial CTG should be performed.

Often on arrival for assessment a woman reports normal movements have resumed. In such cases, if the CTG is normal, on the background of a low-risk pregnancy and if this is the first episode then the woman can be reassured and discharged.

If despite a normal CTG she were to have any risk factors in her pregnancy (for example a small baby, gestational diabetes, hypertension) or if this was not her first episode of reduced fetal movements then a fetal growth and assessment scan should be arranged within 24 hours. If she is still not feeling fetal movements then admission to the unit for serial CTG monitoring is appropriate until a scan can be arranged. Should there be any CTG concerns then these should be acted on appropriately.

Reduced Fetal Movements at Term

Reduced fetal movements at term are an indication for induction of labour (rather than awaiting an ultrasound scan) as the reduced movements may be a sign of ensuing fetal compromise and there is less to be gained from expectant management once the fetus is mature. A discussion with the woman should include explanation of the induction process and the possibility of unsuccessful induction, set against the potential risk of continuing the pregnancy if the fetus is compromised. If the patient declines an induction in this situation then a scan should be still arranged as soon as possible.

 KEY POINTS

- Reduced fetal movements are associated with a higher chance of stillbirth and should be taken seriously despite duration.
- Reduced fetal movements at term are an indication for induction of labour.

CASE 72: ABSENT FETAL MOVEMENTS

History

A 34-year-old woman at 32 weeks and 4 days' gestation in her first pregnancy reports reduced fetal movements. She normally feels the baby move in a regular pattern throughout the day but has not now felt the baby move for the last few hours. She has no significant medical, obstetric or gynaecological history. In this pregnancy she booked at 10 weeks' gestation and all her booking blood tests were normal except that she was discovered not to be immune to rubella and postnatal vaccination was planned. Her 11–14-week scan, nuchal translucency test and anomaly scan were all normal.

Examination

The blood pressure is 137/73 mmHg and pulse 93/min. She is apyrexial. The symphysiofundal height of the uterus is 31 cm and the fetus is breech on examination. The fetal heart is auscultated with hand-held Doppler and no heartbeat is heard. An ultrasound scan is therefore arranged immediately, which confirms the diagnosis of intrauterine fetal death.

? | **QUESTIONS**

- How should this case be managed?
- Are there any factors in the history or examination to indicate the cause of fetal death and what investigations should be performed to establish a possible cause?

DOI: 10.1201/9781003386933-77

ANSWER 72

Immediate Management

The baby needs delivery to avoid the possibility of sepsis or disseminated intravascular coagulopathy developing. This is normally achieved by induction of labour with mifepristone (an antiprogestogen) followed 48 h later by misoprostol (a prostaglandin analogue) to induce contractions. The woman can go home temporarily after the mifepristone.

In labour, adequate analgesia is essential and patient-controlled analgesia (PCA) is useful. Most labour wards have specific suites for bereaved women so they do not have to interact with other newborn babies.

Rarely there are contraindications to vaginal delivery, such as previous caesarean sections, in which case operative delivery may be necessary.

The couple should be seen as soon as possible by a bereavement midwife to discuss the loss, and funeral or cremation plans. Discussion should be had about postmortem examination with a senior obstetrician. Follow-up appointments should be planned to go through the results of any investigations and to discuss plans for future pregnancies if wanted.

Cause of Intrauterine Death

In many cases no cause of intrauterine death is identified. In this history the only potentially significant factor is the lack of rubella immunity. This is unlikely to be significant, but rubella immunoglobulin (IgG) should be checked to exclude recent infection.

The examination is normal except for possibly slightly reduced symphysiofundal height and maternal tachycardia, which may relate to anxiety and should be rechecked.

!   **POSSIBLE CAUSES OF INTRAUTERINE DEATH**

- *Maternal*:
  - Diabetes
  - Infection (e.g. parvovirus, listeria)
  - Thrombophilia (e.g. antiphospholipid syndrome)
- *Fetal*:
  - Chromosomal abnormality (e.g. trisomy)
  - Other genetic abnormality (e.g. Gaucher's disease)
  - Haemolytic disease
  - Cord incident (e.g. 'knot' in cord)
- *Placental*:
  - Placental abruption
  - Uteroplacental insufficiency (e.g. secondary to pre-eclampsia)
  - Postmaturity
- *Unexplained*

INVESTIGATIONS

- *Maternal*:
  - Full blood count and coagulation screen (to exclude disseminated intravascular coagulopathy/thrombocytopenia secondary to fetal death)
  - Random blood glucose and haemoglobin (Hb)A$_{1c}$
  - Kleihauer test (for fetal cells in the maternal circulation, implying significant fetomaternal haemorrhage)
  - Anticardiolipin and lupus anticoagulant (for antiphospholipid syndrome)
- *Fetal*:
  - Swabs for microscopy, culture and sensitivity from the fetus and placenta
  - Skin biopsy for karyotype
  - Postmortem (if agreed by parents)

 KEY POINTS

- Intrauterine death is commonly unexpected and unexplained.
- Induction of labour should be arranged as soon as possible as there is a risk of the development of sepsis or disseminated intravascular coagulopathy.
- Bereavement counselling is one of the most important aspects of care of the woman and family.

History

You are on duty on the labour ward and called to see a 33-year-old woman in labour as the midwife is concerned about the cardiotocograph (CTG).

She is 41 weeks 2 days' gestation and this is her first baby. The pregnancy was uncomplicated until 2 days ago when she developed mild hypertension, without proteinuria. In view of the gestational age a decision was made for induction of labour yesterday. She had 2 mg prostaglandin gel administered into the vagina at 6 pm last night and again at 6 am this morning. Spontaneous rupture of membranes occurred at 10 am today after which contractions commenced.

Examination

Blood pressure is 135/68 mmHg, heart rate 90/min and temperature is 37.1 degrees.

On abdominal palpation the fetus is cephalic, 1/5 palpable and strong contractions are felt. Vaginally the cervix is fully effaced and 6 cm dilated. The fetus is cephalic above ischial spines with mild caput but no moulding. Thin meconium is noted.

🔎 INVESTIGATIONS

The CTG, as shown in Figure 73.1, has demonstrated a similar pattern for approximately 50 min.

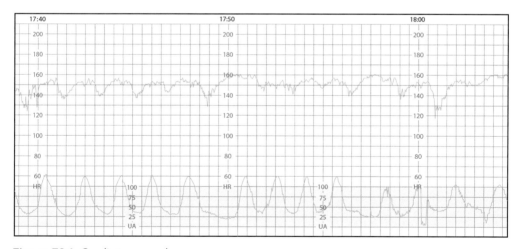

Figure 73.1 Cardiotocograph.

? QUESTIONS

- How would you interpret the CTG?
- How would you manage the patient?

DOI: 10.1201/9781003386933-78

ANSWER 73

The CTG shows a baseline of 155/min with reduced variability (<5/min) and atypical variable decelerations with over 50 per cent of contractions. No accelerations are seen. The CTG is therefore classified as pathological (one red feature and one amber feature, according to National Institute for Health and Clinical Excellence [NICE] guidance). Contractions are 5 in 10.

The classification system for CTG interpretation is outlined in Case 79.

The meconium-stained liquor may be a sign of fetal compromise, but at 41 weeks' gestation meconium may be an incidental finding and is therefore difficult to interpret. Abnormal CTG findings in the presence of meconium are cause for concern as meconium aspiration can occur.

Management

As the CTG is pathological an intervention needs to take place to try to correct the cause – in this case the cause may be hyperstimulation as she is contracting 5 in 10. If not corrected by conservative measures, such as fluids and repositioning of the mother, then delivery needs to be expedited. If the cervix was fully dilated and the head below the ischial spines then instrumental delivery, by ventouse or forceps, would be appropriate. As this is not the case, then immediate delivery by caesarean section is essential. The important points for an emergency caesarean section are:

- The midwife in charge, theatre staff, obstetric consultant, specialist registrar, anaesthetist and paediatrician should be informed.
- The reasons for the proposed procedure should be explained to the woman and informed consent obtained.
- Metoclopramide and omeprazole should be given in case of the need for general anaesthetic.
- Intravenous access is needed with full blood count and group and saves sent.
- A urethral catheter should be inserted.
- The baby should be delivered within a maximum of 60 minutes after the decision.

🔑 **KEY POINTS**

- Atypical variable decelerations with more than 50 per cent of contractions or a single prolonged deceleration for more than 3 min are suggestive of a pathological CTG, and fetal blood sampling or immediate delivery in such cases should be considered urgently.
- CTG interpretation guidelines are published by NICE and should be integrated into all obstetric care in the UK.

CASE 74: PERIPARTUM COLLAPSE

History

A woman aged 28 years is in labour when she suddenly collapses. This is her fourth pregnancy and she has had three previous spontaneous vaginal deliveries at term. This pregnancy has been uncomplicated and she came into the hospital with contractions at 37 weeks and 6 days.

On arrival on the labour ward the fetus was palpated to be normal size, cephalic and 3/5 palpable abdominally. The cervix was 3 cm dilated and the membranes were intact. Blood pressure and urinalysis were normal. Initial auscultation of the fetus was reassuring and the heart rate has continued to be normal (around 140/min) on intermittent auscultation.

Five minutes ago spontaneous rupture of membranes occurred during a contraction, with a large gush of clear fluid from the vagina. The woman reported an urge to push at that stage and then became confused and disorientated saying that she could not breathe and was going to die. Immediately following this she collapsed.

Examination

The woman is unconscious and unrousable to painful stimuli. The blood pressure is 98/40 mmHg and heart rate 120/min. The oxygen saturation is 86 per cent on air and respiratory rate 24/min. The heart sounds are normal but on chest examination there are inspiratory crackles throughout the chest.

The abdomen is soft with intermittent contractions continuing, and in fact the fetal head is now visible at the perineum. There is no vaginal bleeding.

> **?** | **QUESTIONS**
>
> - What is the likely diagnosis and differential diagnosis?
> - How would you manage this woman?

DOI: 10.1201/9781003386933-79

ANSWER 74

The diagnosis is likely to be an amniotic fluid embolism.

Differential diagnoses include:

- Pulmonary embolism
- Myocardial infarction
- Vasovagal episode

The factors leading to the diagnosis of amniotic fluid embolism rather than one of the differentials are the history of sudden collapse without preceding chest pain, and the fact that this occurred around the time of rupture of membranes. Amniotic fluid embolism is also often preceded by premonitory symptoms, restlessness, confusion or cyanosis. A vasovagal episode is very unlikely as this is usually associated with bradycardia and would not account for the chest signs or decreased oxygen saturation.

Amniotic fluid embolism occurs when amniotic fluid enters the maternal circulation. This is usually during labour but can occur with maternal trauma or very occasionally after delivery. It is rare (estimated to occur in between 1 in 8000 and 1 in 80,000 pregnancies), unpredictable, sudden and commonly fatal (between 30 and 86 per cent reported fatality rates). Women who die tend to do so within an hour or so of becoming unwell, having developed acute hypoxia, coagulopathy and cardiac arrest.

Management

The baby should be delivered immediately as this will facilitate more effective resuscitation of the mother. In this case a simple forceps delivery should be performed. If the baby was not deliverable vaginally then immediate caesarean section should be performed. Massive postpartum haemorrhage is very likely and syntocinon infusion should be commenced with further postpartum haemorrhage strategies such as ergometrine, carboprost, tranexamic acid, embolization or hysterectomy anticipated. There is no definitive treatment for amniotic fluid embolism and the management is purely supportive.

!   RESUSCITATION OF THE MOTHER AFTER SUSPECTED AMNIOTIC FLUID EMBOLISM

- Insertion of two large-bore intravenous cannulae
- Request for full blood count, urea and electrolytes, clotting profile, fibrin-degradation products
- Crossmatch 6 units blood and have platelets and fresh-frozen plasma available
- One hundred per cent oxygen by bag and mask initially with intubation by the anaesthetist as soon as possible
- Volume expansion with crystalloid fluids
- Transfer to intensive care unit as soon as possible

🔑   KEY POINTS

- Sudden collapse in labour is an obstetric emergency.
- The diagnosis of amniotic fluid embolism is usually made postmortem.

History

A 32-year-old woman is brought into the delivery suite by ambulance 6 days following a vaginal delivery at 39 weeks' gestation. The pregnancy and labour had been unremarkable and the placenta was delivered by controlled cord traction.

Following delivery the woman had been discharged home after 6 h. She reported that the lochia had been heavy for the first 2 days but that it had then settled to less than a period. However today she had suddenly felt crampy abdominal pain and felt a gush of fluid, followed by very heavy bleeding. The blood has soaked through clothes and she has passed large clots, which she describes as the size of her fist. She feels dizzy when she stands up and is nauseated.

Examination

She is pale with cool and clammy extremities. She is also drowsy. Her blood pressure is 105/50 mmHg and heart rate is 112/min. On abdominal palpation there is minimal tenderness but the uterus is palpable approximately 6 cm above the symphysis pubis.

Speculum examination reveals large clots of blood in the vagina. When these are removed, the cervix is seen to be open.

 QUESTIONS

- What is the diagnosis?
- What is your immediate and subsequent management?
- Should an ultrasound scan be requested?

DOI: 10.1201/9781003386933-80

ANSWER 75

The diagnosis is secondary postpartum haemorrhage.

> **! POSTPARTUM HAEMORRHAGE**
>
> Postpartum haemorrhage is defined as the loss of more than 500 mL of blood vaginally following delivery. Primary postpartum haemorrhage is within 24 h. Secondary postpartum haemorrhage occurs between 24 h and 6 weeks following delivery.

> **! COMMON CAUSES OF POSTPARTUM HAEMORRHAGE**
>
> - Retained placental tissue (products of conception)
> - Vaginal trauma
> - Endometrial infection
> - Coagulopathy (e.g. following placental abruption)
> - Uterine atony

Immediate Management

This woman is in hypovolaemic shock and needs immediate resuscitation. Two wide-bore cannulae should be inserted and blood sent for full blood count, urea and electrolytes, clotting and crossmatch of 4 units, with further red cells, platelets or fresh-frozen plasma requested depending on further evaluation and blood results. Immediate intravenous fluid should be administered.

The uterus should be rubbed suprapubically, and if this fails to reduce the bleeding immediately then bimanual compression commenced, pending administration of 500 mg ergometrine, 1g tranexamic acid and commencing a syntocinon infusion. These measures stem the blood loss and aid immediate resuscitation while the diagnosis is investigated. A urinary catheter should be inserted to allow close fluid balance monitoring and renal function; this also helps with contraction of the uterus. The anaesthetist and senior obstetrician should be called urgently.

Subsequent Management

The fact that the cervix is open is considered pathognomonic of retained tissue. In this situation, an ultrasound is not indicated to determine management, and evacuation of retained products of conception should be arranged once the woman has been resuscitated and blood is available. This should however be carried out under ultrasound guidance.

In view of the haemodynamic instability, general anaesthetic is preferred. Intravenous antibiotics should be given. The woman should be monitored initially in a high-dependency setting until clinically and haematologically stable.

Although she may have had a coagulopathy at admission, she is still at high risk of venous thromboembolism as she has had a postpartum haemorrhage and has undergone anaesthetic. Thromboembolic stockings and heparin should therefore be administered postoperatively.

> **🔑 KEY POINTS**
>
> - Postpartum women with retained products of conception become very ill very quickly.
> - Once the diagnosis is made intravenous antibiotics and urgent evacuation of the uterus are necessary.

CASE 76: PERINEAL WOUND INFECTION

History

A 34-year-old woman presents to the obstetric triage unit with increasing perineal pain 5 days following a forceps delivery.

Her pregnancy had been classified as high risk in light of the BMI of 37 kg/m^2 and pre-existing type 2 diabetes. Because of the diabetes she underwent an induction of labour at 39 weeks' gestation. The first stage was uncomplicated and in the second stage she pushed for 2 hours and then had a forceps delivery in theatre with an episiotomy which was sutured.

She reports increasing perineal pain over the last 2 days and it has become very sore to pass urine. Her lochia is normal but she has noticed there to be some smelly discharge also on her pads. She does not report any fever and says that she feels systemically well although tired.

Examination

On examination she is clearly in discomfort sitting upright but this improves on lying on her side. Her heart rate is 80/min, temperature is 36.5 degrees, blood pressure 120/70 mmHg and respiratory rate is 12/min. Her abdomen is soft and non-tender with her uterus palpable midway between the umbilicus and symphysis pubis. Her lochia seems appropriate to postnatal day 5. The episiotomy wound is gaping open 1 cm with obvious pus around the sutures.

Blood Results

INVESTIGATIONS

		Normal Range
Haemoglobin	120 g/L	110–140 g/L
White cell count	12 × 10⁹/L	6–10 × 10⁹/L
Neutrophils	8 × 10⁹/L	2.5–7 × 10⁹/L
Platelets	350 × 10⁹/L	150–400 × 10⁹/L
Sodium	135 mmol/L	130–140 mmol/L
Potassium	3.4 mmol/L	3.3–4.1 mmol/L
Urea	6 mmol/L	2.4–4.3 mmol/L
Creatinine	80 mmol/L	34–82 mmol/L
C-reactive protein	70 mg/L	<5 mg/L

? QUESTIONS

- What is the diagnosis?
- Could this have been prevented?
- How would you manage this patient now?

DOI: 10.1201/9781003386933-81

ANSWER 76

This woman has a perineal wound infection following an instrumental delivery. This is a common complication following approximately 10 per cent of women after vaginal delivery. It is therefore very important to give women adequate advice following any perineal trauma about how to care for the area, to help promote healing and prevent infection.

> **! ADVICE FOR WOMEN AFTER OBSTETRIC PERINEAL TRAUMA**
>
> - Try to keep the area clean and dry.
>   - Shower (if possible) or bath once or twice a day.
>   - Allow the water to get to the affected area and dry by patting with a clean dry towel or using a hairdryer on a cool setting.
>   - After going to the toilet, pour warm water over the vaginal area to rinse it.
>   - Wipe from front to back after opening bowels.
>   - Try and keep the wound exposed sometimes during the day by lying down and removing underwear when possible.
> - Change sanitary pads frequently.
> - Use simple analgesia as needed – paracetamol and ibuprofen (if no contraindications) are safe with breast-feeding.
> - Apply ice packs to the area to help with pain.

Instrumental deliveries are a risk factor for perineal wound infection and it is now standard to give one intravenous dose of antibiotic following any instrumental delivery. This woman was also at an increased risk of developing an infection due to her diabetes and raised BMI.

If any sutures are easily removed this should also be considered to aid healing. A wound swab should be taken for culture and sensitivity and the wound should be cleaned with saline and then left to heal by secondary intention. This is because resuturing infected tissue can make the situation worse.

An oral broad spectrum treatment antibiotic (such as co-amoxiclav) for 7 days should be started with a review after 3–5 days to ensure improvement. If the woman showed signs of systemic infection (such as fever, rigors or vomiting) then she should be admitted for blood cultures and intravenous antibiotics.

Once healed, if the woman is unhappy with appearance of the wound or has ongoing pain then she should be offered review in a gynaecology clinic 3 months postnatally for discussion of perineal refashioning (perineorrhaphy).

> **🔑 KEY POINTS**
>
> - Perineal wound infections are a common complication and women can present to a variety of healthcare settings.
> - Oral broad-spectrum antibiotics are appropriate if not systemically unwell.
> - All women should be given one dose of intravenous antibiotic following instrumental delivery.

History

A 31-year-old woman is admitted with contractions at 40 weeks' gestation. This is her fourth pregnancy, having had two terminations approximately 10 years ago and an elective caesarean section for breech presentation 3 years ago.

During this pregnancy she has had an amniocentesis because of a high estimated risk for Down's syndrome at 11–14-week scan. However a normal karyotype result was reported and subsequent fetal echocardiography was normal. In view of her previous caesarean section she was seen by the obstetric consultant in the antenatal clinic at 28 weeks to discuss mode of delivery. After counselling, a plan was agreed to aim for a vaginal delivery.

She was admitted with spontaneous rupture of membranes after which she had begun to contract irregularly. The contractions became stronger and more regular over the next 2 h after admission and she requested an epidural. Vaginal examination was performed and the cervix was found to be 4 cm dilated. The head was in the occipitotransverse position, 1 cm above the level of the ischial spines. There was a small amount of caput and moulding.

An epidural was sited and an indwelling urinary catheter inserted. Three hours later the woman reported more severe pain which did not disappear between contractions. At that time approximately 200 mL of fresh blood was seen coming from the vagina.

Examination

Her heart rate is 105/min and blood pressure 105/58 mmHg. The woman feels warm and well perfused. The abdomen is soft and the uterus is also soft but very tender, with easy palpation of fetal parts. On vaginal examination the cervix is 6 cm dilated and the fetal head feels high in the pelvis and poorly applied to the cervix. The catheter contains blood-stained urine.

| INVESTIGATIONS |

The cardiotocograph (CTG) is described below and shown in Figure 77.1.

CTG report:

- Fetal heart rate initially 150/min with variability 20/min
- Sudden prolonged fall in fetal heart rate to 80/min
- No accelerations
- Loss of uterine activity at time of fetal bradycardia

? QUESTIONS

- What is the likely diagnosis?
- How would you manage this patient?
- What are the possible further complications for this patient?

DOI: 10.1201/9781003386933-82

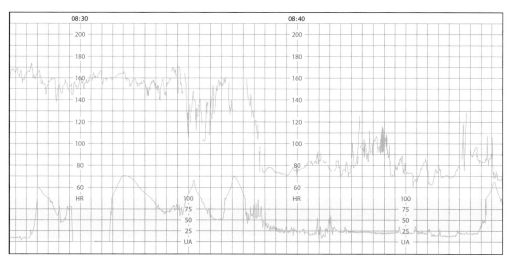

Figure 77.1 Cardiotocograph.

ANSWER 77

The CTG shows that the contractions have stopped. This appearance can be due to the pressure transducer losing contact with the patient, but in this case the combination of other factors and the fact that the uterus is soft on palpation suggests that the contractions really have suddenly stopped.

The diagnosis is of uterine rupture. The constant pain, vaginal bleeding, sudden loss of contractions, change in CTG, loss of presenting part in the pelvis, easy palpation of fetal parts and haematuria are all classic features. Uterine rupture is thought to occur in up to 1 in 200 labours following caesarean section. It is more common when labour is induced with prostaglandins or augmented with oxytocin infusion, but may occur even in an apparently 'normal' labour such as this. Uterine rupture may very rarely occur in women without previous caesarean section, either because of previous surgery such as myomectomy, with trauma or spontaneously. The major risk factor for uterine rupture is previous caesarean section.

General resuscitation measures should be commenced immediately:

- Large-bore intravenous access
- Full blood count, coagulation test
- 6-unit crossmatch requested
- Intravenous fluids

The emergency theatre team, senior obstetrician and paediatrician should be summoned and the woman transferred to theatre immediately for laparotomy, which may need to be under general anaesthetic as the epidural is unlikely to be adequate for laparotomy within a few minutes.

At laparotomy, the fetus should be delivered from the abdomen and the placenta removed. It may be possible to repair the uterine defect. However, if bleeding is substantial then other measures may need to be employed such as a B-Lynch haemostatic suture or even hysterectomy.

If the uterus is preserved, then any future pregnancies should be very closely monitored with elective delivery by caesarean section at 37 weeks' gestation.

!   **COMPLICATIONS OF UTERINE RUPTURE**

- *Fetal*:
  - Death
  - Cerebral palsy from hypoxic brain injury
- *Maternal*:
  - Postpartum haemorrhage
  - Hysterectomy
  - Coagulopathy

    KEY POINTS

- Dehiscence of a previous caesarean section scar can range from a dramatic to subtle presentation.
- Change in CTG pattern, persistent abdominal pain, cessation of contractions, maternal tachycardia or haematuria should alert the clinician to the possibility of uterine rupture.

CASE 78: LABOUR

History

A midwife is concerned about a cardiotocograph (CTG) on the labour ward. The woman is 42 years old and had an elective caesarean section 3 years ago for twins. After counselling, she decided to opt for a vaginal delivery in this pregnancy. She is now at a gestational age of 38 weeks and 1 day and presented to the labour ward an hour ago. She was found to have contractions, three in 10 min lasting 50 s each. There has been no reported rupture of membranes.

At the time of arrival, examination revealed a symphysiofundal height of 39 cm, cephalic presentation and 3/5 palpable abdominally. Vaginal examination revealed intact membranes with the head 1 cm above the ischial spines, occipitoanterior position and the cervix 5 cm dilated.

She was commenced on continuous CTG monitoring (because of the previous caesarean section), which showed an initial baseline rate of 135/min, good variability, accelerations and no decelerations.

Twenty minutes ago spontaneous rupture of membranes occurred with clear liquor leaking.

🔍 **INVESTIGATIONS**

The CTG is shown in Figure 78.1.

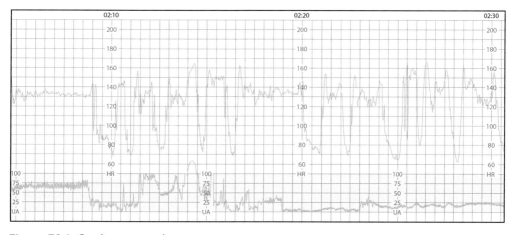

Figure 78.1 Cardiotocograph.

? **QUESTIONS**

- Describe and classify the CTG.
- What are the possible causes for this CTG pattern?
- What should be your subsequent management?

DOI: 10.1201/9781003386933-83

ANSWER 78

The CTG shows a baseline rate of 130/min and variability of 15/min. There are atypical variable decelerations to approximately 70/min lasting 30–90 s. There are no accelerations but there is 'shouldering' before and after the decelerations, a sign of the fetus increasing its heart rate in response to the increased blood flow after the deceleration. The fetal heartbeat is only just recovering to the baseline between decelerations.

This CTG is unsatisfactory because the tocometer is not registering contractions.

Management

In this situation, the recent history of spontaneous rupture of membranes indicates immediate vaginal assessment to rule out cord prolapse as the cause of the suddenly abnormal CTG. This would be a classic presentation for cord prolapse, though the condition itself is very rare.

Much more commonly variable decelerations are caused by cord compression (against the uterine wall or, for example, compression by the fetal hand).

If, as is normally the case, the cord is not palpable and the baby is not easily deliverable by instrumental delivery, then further assessment of the full clinical picture is warranted. Specifically in this case assessing for signs of uterine rupture is vital as she has a scar on her uterus from a previous delivery. A good indication of fetal wellbeing is an acceleration noted on the CTG when the fetal scalp is stimulated.

In this case the CTG was deemed pathological but the cervix was fully dilated and the head low on examination, with good fetal response to scalp stimulation, and she rapidly progressed to a vaginal delivery of a live infant in good condition 15 minutes later with pushing.

 KEY POINT

- CTGs are classified according to national guidelines (as shown in Tables 78.1 and 78.2).

Table 78.1 Definition of Normal, Suspicious and Pathological FHR Traces

Category	Definition
Normal	All four features (baseline rate, variability, decelerations and acceleration) are classified as reassuring
Suspicious	One feature is classified as non-reassuring and the remaining features classified as reassuring
Pathological	Two or more features are classified as non-reassuring or one or more classified as abnormal

Table 78.2 Classification of FHR Trace Features

Feature	Baseline (Beats/Min)	Variability (Beats/Min)	Decelerations	Accelerations
Reassuring	110–160	≥5	None or early Variable decelerations with no concerning characteristics for less than 90 minutes	Present
Non-reassuring	100–109 161–180	<5 for 40–90 min	Variable decelerations with no concerning characteristics for over 90 mins OR Variable decelerations with any concerning characteristics in up to 50% of contractions for 30 mins or more OR Variable decelerations with any concerning characteristics in over 50% of contractions for less than 30 minutes OR Late decelerations in over 50% of contractions for less than 30 minutes with no clinical risk factors such as vaginal bleeding or significant meconium	The absence of accelerations with otherwise normal trace is of uncertain significance
Abnormal	<100 >180 Sinusoidal pattern ≥10min	<5 for 90 min	Variable decelerations with any concerning characteristics in over 50% contractions for 30 minutes (or less if clinical risk factors) OR Late decelerations for 30 minutes (or less if clinical risk factors) OR Acute bradycardia or a single prolonged deceleration lasting 3 minutes or more	

Source: NICE Clinical guideline CG190 (February 2017).

CASE 79: LABOUR

History

A 22-year-old woman in her second pregnancy has arrived on the labour ward at 38 weeks 3 days. She had a vaginal delivery 18 months ago. This pregnancy has been complicated by persistent vomiting until 20 weeks and more recently by anaemia. She reports contractions commencing approximately 4 h ago. She took paracetamol at home and tried to relieve the pain with a bath, but now feels she cannot cope with the pain.

She had a show 2 days ago but has had no bleeding since then and has not noticed any vaginal leak. She has felt the baby moving normally all day.

Examination

The blood pressure is 110/58 mmHg and heart rate is 98/min. The fetal presentation is cephalic with 2/5 palpable abdominally. Uterine contractions are palpable and the uterus is non-irritable. On vaginal examination the cervix is 5 cm dilated and the head is 1 cm above the ischial spines. The fetal position is right occipitotransverse with mild caput and moulding. The membranes are intact but rupture spontaneously during examination, with clear liquor draining.

The woman requests an epidural for pain relief and is therefore commenced on continuous cardiotocograph monitoring. After 20 min you are called in to review the situation.

🔍 **INVESTIGATIONS**

The CTG as you walk in is shown in Figure 79.1.

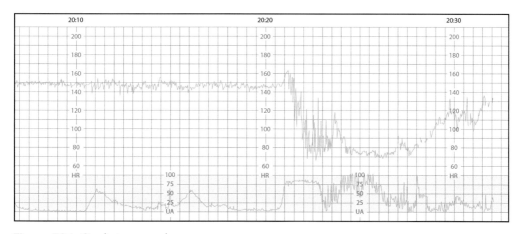

Figure 79.1 Cardiotocograph.

❓ **QUESTIONS**

- Describe the CTG.
- What are the possible causes of this CTG?
- What management would be appropriate now?

DOI: 10.1201/9781003386933-84

ANSWER 79

CTG Interpretation

The initial 15 min of the CTG shows a baseline of 145/min with normal variability (12/min) and no visible accelerations or decelerations. Following this there is a drop in fetal heart rate to 70/min for 7 min before gradual recovery to 125/min. Contractions are 2 in 10 until the tocograph becomes unreadable.

This is a previously low-risk pregnancy and this CTG shows a fetal bradycardia (reduction in baseline heart rate to below 100/min). In many cases no cause is identified, but some potential causes are shown in the following list.

> **! CAUSES OF FETAL BRADYCARDIA**
>
> - Placental abruption
> - Uterine rupture
> - Maternal hypotension (e.g. after epidural insertion)
> - Bleeding vasa praevia

Management

The 'rule of 3s' should be employed in managing this woman:

- If the deceleration has not recovered at 3 min call for help.
- If the deceleration has not recovered at 6 min transfer to theatre and prepare for immediate delivery.
- If the deceleration has not recovered at 9 min deliver immediately by category one ('crash') caesarean section (if immediate instrumental vaginal delivery is not possible). This will usually involve general anaesthetic unless an effective spinal anaesthetic is achievable by an experienced anaesthetist in a similar time.

The labour ward theatre emergency team should be called (including anaesthetist, obstetric registrar, paediatrician, midwife in charge, theatre staff) and the woman transferred to the operating theatre. On occasion the bradycardia recovers as preparation is underway for the caesarean, in which case the plan may be reviewed. Otherwise the baby should be delivered immediately.

In this case the bradycardia did not recover and the baby was delivered within 12 min of the decision being made. No cause was found for the bradycardia at caesarean section.

>   **INVESTIGATIONS**
>
> The umbilical artery cord blood analysis at delivery was:
>
> | | Artery | Vein |
> | --- | --- | --- |
> | pH | 7.06 | 7.23 |
> | pCO_2 | 8.20 mmHg | 6.30 mmHg |
> | Base excess | −6.4 mmol/L | −5.2 mmol/L |

The baby initially made poor respiratory effort and had a heart rate less than 100/min, but recovered quickly with drying and warming. The Apgar score for the baby was 5 at 1 min and 9 at 5 min.

 KEY POINTS

- A prolonged bradycardia (>6 min) is an indication to transfer a woman to theatre for consideration of immediate delivery if the heart rate has not then recovered by 9 min.
- There is no place for a fetal blood sample in the management of fetal bradycardia.
- A cause is not always found for an abnormal CTG.

CASE 80: PAIN AND FEVER IN PREGNANCY

History

A woman aged 26 years is referred by her general practitioner. She is 36 weeks' gestation in her fourth pregnancy, having had one miscarriage and two term vaginal deliveries.

In this pregnancy she has been seen twice in the day assessment unit, the first time at 31 weeks for an episode of vaginal bleeding for which no cause was attributed. The second time was at 35 weeks after she awoke with damp bed sheets. No liquor had been detected on speculum examination at the time and she was discharged. For the last 2 days she has been feeling generally unwell with a fever, decreased appetite and a headache as well as abdominal discomfort. She reports the baby moving less than normal for the last few days.

She has not noticed any vaginal bleeding but her discharge has been more than normal and there is an offensive odour to it.

Examination

Her temperature is 37.8 degrees, blood pressure 106/68 mmHg and heart rate 109/min. On abdominal palpation symphysiofundal height is 34 cm and the fetus is cephalic with 3/5 palpable. There is generalized uterine tenderness and irritability. On speculum examination the cervix is closed and a green/grey discharge is seen within the vagina.

🔍 INVESTIGATIONS		
		Normal Range for Pregnancy
Haemoglobin	109 g/L	110–140 g/L
Mean cell volume	80 fL	74.4–95.6 fL
White cell count	17.3×10^9/L	$6-16 \times 10^9$/L
Platelets	327×10^9/L	$150-400 \times 10^9$/L
C-reactive protein	68 mg/L	<5 mg/L

The cardiotocograph (CTG) is shown in Figure 80.1.

DOI: 10.1201/9781003386933-85

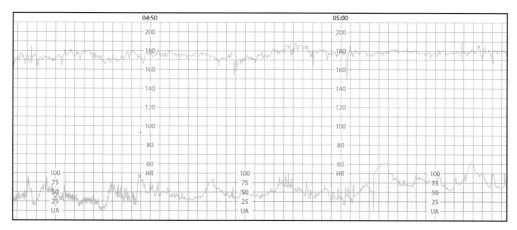

Figure 80.1 Cardiotocograph.

? | **QUESTIONS**

- What is the diagnosis?
- How should this woman be managed?

ANSWER 80

The diagnosis is of chorioamnionitis secondary to prolonged preterm rupture of membranes. Although spontaneous rupture of membranes was not confirmed at the previous attendance at 35 weeks, it seems probable that in fact this did occur at that time. Use of a test like AmniSure Rupture of Membranes test (which detects placental alpha microglobulin-1 protein) could have assisted in determining this. Ascending organisms have subsequently colonized the uterus and resulted in infection. The result is a maternal systemic reaction causing the patient's symptoms and signs: tachycardia, tenderness, leucocytosis and raised C-reactive protein.

The fetus is also affected as shown by the fetal tachycardia.

Chorioamnionitis is a significant cause of both fetal and maternal morbidity and mortality, and should be treated as an obstetric emergency.

Management should be instigated immediately. Initial microbial specimens should be obtained from high vaginal swab and maternal blood cultures.

Intravenous broad-spectrum antibiotic should be commenced to cover both anaerobic and aerobic organisms. Intravenous fluids should be commenced to counter the effects of vasodilatation and pyrexia, and because the woman is unable to drink adequately. Paracetamol should be given regularly for the pyrexia and abdominal discomfort.

The baby needs delivery ideally by induction of labour – women with chorioamnionitis often labour rapidly. Risks of caesarean section in the presence of infection are significant in terms of bleeding, uterine atony and disseminated intravascular coagulopathy. However continuous CTG should be employed and immediate caesarean section performed if the fetus shows signs of deterioration.

After delivery, the baby will be reviewed by the paediatrician and given a septic screen and potentially a course of intravenous antibiotics.

KEY POINTS

- Chorioamnionitis is a significant cause of fetal and maternal morbidity and must be managed aggressively with antibiotics and induction of labour.
- An uncomplicated fetal tachycardia should be managed with fluids and paracetamol to the mother, with antibiotics if infection is suspected.
- Delivery should be expedited if any other concerning CTG features develop.

CASE 81: HEADACHE IN PREGNANCY

History

A 32-year-old woman who is 34 weeks' gestation has felt generally unwell for 24 h. She has a headache and has noticed odd visual symptoms such as 'wobbling' of objects. She initially felt that she had a viral infection but the symptoms are worsening and she thought she should get 'checked out'.

She has epigastric discomfort and nausea. Her legs have been swollen for some weeks but now her hands and face are puffy. The baby has been moving normally and there is no lower abdominal pain and no bleeding or abnormal discharge.

She booked in the pregnancy at 10 weeks with a blood pressure of 107/60 mmHg. Booking blood tests and 12- and 20-week ultrasound scans were normal.

Examination

Her blood pressure is 140/85 mmHg and pulse rate 98/min. There is moderate oedema to the knees and she also appears digitally and facially oedematous. The fundi are normal.

On abdominal palpation there is mild right upper quadrant and epigastric tenderness. The uterus is not tender and symphysiofundal height measures 33 cm. The fetus is cephalic and free, with fetal parts easily felt on palpation. Patellar reflexes are normal.

🔍 INVESTIGATIONS

		Normal Range for Pregnancy
Haemoglobin	93 g/L	110–140 g/L
Packed cell volume	42%	31–38%
Mean cell volume	81 fL	74.4–95.6 fL
White cell count	6.0×10^9/L	$6–16 \times 10^9$/L
Platelets	97×10^9/L	$150–400 \times 10^9$/L
Sodium	139 mmol/L	130–140 mmol/L
Potassium	4.2 mmol/L	3.3–4.1 mmol/L
Urea	4 mmol/L	2.4–4.3 mmol/L
Creatinine	83 mmol/L	34–82 mmol/L
Alanine transaminase	172 IU/L	6–32 IU/L
Alkaline phosphatase	238 IU/L	30–300 IU/L
Gamma glutamyl transaminase	26 IU/L	5–43 IU/L
Bilirubin	37 mmol/L	3–14 mmol/L
Albumin	26 g/dL	28–37 g/dL
Urate	0.38 mmol/L	0.14–0.38 mmol/L

Urinalysis: Protein ++

❓ QUESTIONS

- What is the likely diagnosis?
- How would you further investigate and manage this patient?

DOI: 10.1201/9781003386933-86

ANSWER 81

The diagnosis is HELLP syndrome (haemolysis, elevated liver enzymes and low platelets).

HELLP syndrome is part of the spectrum of pre-eclampsia, and is a serious condition with a relatively high maternal mortality (1 per cent) and perinatal mortality (up to 60 per cent). Maternal complications include placental abruption, renal failure, liver failure and disseminated intravascular coagulopathy (DIC). Fetal complications arise from prematurity, abruption and uteroplacental insufficiency.

The diagnosis is made on the blood test results showing the haematological and biochemical features of HELLP syndrome. In this case there is also evidence of pre-eclampsia. However these clinical features do not need to be present to make the diagnosis of HELLP syndrome.

HELLP syndrome may present antenatally or in the first few days postpartum.

The symptom of epigastric or right upper quadrant pain should always raise suspicion in a pregnant woman, as it is a sign of liver capsule stretching and may precede liver rupture.

Investigation and Management

The woman needs urgent delivery as the condition improves only once the pregnancy has ended. This may be vaginal, with regular monitoring of the blood test results and proteinuria every 6 h. Hourly blood pressure should be recorded or more frequently if it is outside target range.

A clotting screen is indicated to assess for risk of severe bleeding at delivery.

Vaginal delivery is optimal, assuming the fetal wellbeing is not in question. However if the cervix is unfavourable and the woman is nulliparous then caesarean section may be considered, bearing in mind the associated increased risk of bleeding.

Fetal wellbeing should be checked with cardiotocography and if available ultrasound for growth, liquor volume and umbilical artery Doppler (although this should not delay delivery). The fetal parts being easily palpable may be suggestive of oligohydramnios from uteroplacental insufficiency.

Steroids should be administered to reduce the chance of respiratory distress syndrome, though there may be insufficient time before delivery for them to be effective.

Postnatally the woman should be closely monitored in hospital in a high dependency unit, with supportive care and involvement of the internal medicine team, until blood results start to normalize. She should remain in hospital for up to 5 days as the condition may deteriorate before recovery. Once recovery occurs it is usually complete, but there is an increased risk of pre-eclampsia (and possibly HELLP syndrome) in subsequent pregnancies. This risk can be reduced by commencing aspirin before 16 weeks' gestation.

 KEY POINT

- HELLP syndrome is a very serious condition and requires urgent delivery.

CASE 82: PROLONGED PREGNANCY

History

A 27-year-old primigravid woman is seen in the antenatal clinic at 41 weeks 2 days' gestation.

This pregnancy was conceived naturally and 12-week ultrasound scan confirmed the estimated due date. All routine investigations and monitoring during the pregnancy have been unremarkable.

She reports the baby moving regularly and although she reports having Braxton Hicks contractions, she has had no symptoms or signs of labour.

Examination

The blood pressure is 116/64 mmHg. The urinalysis shows no proteinuria.

The symphysiofundal height is 39 cm. Presentation is cephalic with 2/5 of the head palpable.

The fetal heart is auscultated at 148/min and an acceleration is heard during auscultation.

? | **QUESTIONS**

- How will you counsel this woman about the potential advantages and disadvantages of induction of labour?
- Assuming the decision is made to proceed with induction of labour, outline the process.

DOI: 10.1201/9781003386933-87

ANSWER 82

Prolonged pregnancy, defined as pregnancy continuing beyond 42 weeks' gestation, occurs in 5–10 per cent of women. Prolonged pregnancy is associated with an increased risk of stillbirth, though the absolute risk of this remains low (2–3/1000). Induction of labour for prolonged pregnancy ('post dates') is recommended between 41 and 42 weeks' gestation.

Advantages

Reduced risk of stillbirth associated with prolonged pregnancy – the relative risk of stillbirth from induction of labour after 41 weeks (versus expectant management) is 0.30.

Some women express the wish to deliver soon after 40 weeks because of discomfort, anxiety or social reasons.

Disadvantages

The following risks are associated with induction of labour:

- Uterine hyperstimulation (1–5 per cent).
- Failed induction (15 per cent) – may require repeat induction process or caesarean section.
- Induction of labour can be a prolonged process – sometimes taking more than 24 h for labour to be established.
- Approximately 500 women need to undergo induction of labour to prevent one baby death.
- There is some evidence that induced labour is associated with greater analgesia requirement than spontaneous labour.

Process of Induction of Labour

Membrane Sweep

Membrane sweep after 40 weeks' gestation reduces the need for induction of labour (relative risk 0.59), with eight women needing to undergo membrane sweep to prevent one formal induction of labour. Membrane sweeping can be repeated and probably works by causing local release of prostaglandin.

Prostaglandin

Vaginal prostaglandin E2 (PGE2) is the usual agent used for induction of labour. Typically a slow-release PGE2 tablet/gel is used, or a controlled-release pessary, which has the advantage of being removable if hyperstimulation occurs.

The decision to give prostaglandin or perform amniotomy is based on the modified Bishop score (see Table 82.1). The Bishop score should then be reassessed 6 h after vaginal PGE2 insertion, or 24 h after vaginal PGE2 controlled-release pessary insertion, to monitor progress.

Mechanical Dilatation of the Cervix

Some mechanical (non-pharmacological) methods are available to cause cervical dilatation. These include an intracervical balloon catheter or an intracervical osmotic hygroscopic dilator which acts as a sponge to draw moisture from the cervix, both causing sufficient dilatation to allow for amniotomy. These methods are used routinely in women with previous caesarean sections to avoid the increased risk of rupture from prostaglandin methods.

Table 82.1 **The Modified Bishop Score**

Cervical Feature	Modified Bishop Score			
	0	*1*	*2*	*3*
Dilation (cm)	<1	1–2	2–4	>4
Length of cervix (cm)	>4	2–4	1–2	<1
Station (relative to ischial spines)	−3	−2	−1/0	+1/+2
Consistency	Firm	Average	Soft	–
Position	Posterior	Mid/anterior	–	–

Amniotomy

Artificial rupture of the membranes is performed once the Bishop score is 6 or more. In some women, particularly multigravida women, it may be possible to perform amniotomy at presentation, thus preventing the need for prostaglandins. Most women however will need at least one dose of prostaglandin prior to amniotomy.

Oxytocin

Intravenous oxytocin infusion should be started after amniotomy. The dose is titrated against the fetal heart rate and contractions, with the aim of achieving four strong contractions every 10 min.

Fetal Monitoring during Induction of Labour

Electronic fetal monitoring (EFM) should be carried out before and after either insertion of prostaglandin or amniotomy. Following this, intermittent auscultation is reasonable until either labour is established or oxytocin is commenced, from which point continuous EFM is required.

Expectant Management of Prolonged Pregnancy

In a woman who declines induction of labour for prolonged pregnancy beyond 42 weeks' gestation, increased antenatal monitoring consisting of at least twice-weekly cardiotocography and ultrasound estimation of maximum amniotic pool depth should be offered although it should be communicated that this does not guarantee the wellbeing of the baby.

 KEY POINTS

- Induction of labour is recommended between 41 and 42 weeks' gestation to reduce the risk of stillbirth.
- The relative risk of stillbirth is 0.3 for induction of labour after 41 weeks (versus expectant management).
- Prostaglandin gel or pessary is the most common induction agent, but induction may also be achieved by membrane sweep, mechanical methods or amniotomy alone.

CASE 83: PAIN IN PREGNANCY

History

A 28-year-old nulliparous woman is admitted to the labour ward at 31 weeks and 6 days' gestation, with abdominal pain.

In this pregnancy she has had chronic low back pain for which she has been under the care of a physiotherapist. She has also been treated for confirmed urinary tract infections on two occasions. She underwent two large-loop excisions of the transformation zone (LLETZ) procedures some years ago. Since then her smears have been normal, the most recent being 10 months ago.

Yesterday she noticed an increase in her discharge with some dark vaginal bleeding and abdominal discomfort. She thought the symptoms may have been related to something she had eaten but she now feels intermittent abdominal pain every few minutes, with no pain in between episodes. Fetal movements are normal.

There is no history of leaking of liquor. She has urinary frequency, though this has not worsened recently. She is always constipated.

Examination

The woman is apyrexial with blood pressure 109/60 mmHg and heart rate 96/min. Symphysiofundal height is 30 cm and moderate contractions are palpated lasting approximately 35 s. The fetus is breech on palpation and the presenting part feels engaged.

No liquor is visible on speculum examination. On vaginal examination the cervix is effaced and 3 cm dilated, with the breech felt –2 cm above the ischial spines and membranes intact.

 INVESTIGATIONS

Cardiotocograph (CTG):

- Baseline rate 145/min, variability normal (15/min)
- Accelerations present
- No decelerations observed
- Uterine activity recorded 3 in 10

? **QUESTIONS**

- What is the diagnosis?
- What factors predispose to this?
- How would you manage this woman?

DOI: 10.1201/9781003386933-88

ANSWER 83

The woman is in premature labour – she has regular painful contractions (as confirmed by the history, palpation and uterine activity demonstrated on CTG) and the cervix is effaced and dilated.

In this history the possible risk factors are the LLETZ procedures and urinary tract infections, raising the possibility that she could be in premature labour due to a further untreated urinary tract infection. However, many women in premature labour have no obvious risk factors.

! RISK FACTORS FOR PREMATURE LABOUR

- *Maternal*:
  - History of premature delivery
  - Previous cervical surgery
  - Young maternal age
  - Illegal drug use and smoking
  - Chorioamnionitis
  - Pre-eclampsia
  - Polyhydramnios
  - Sepsis
- *Fetal*:
  - Intrauterine growth retardation
  - Congenital abnormality
  - Multiple pregnancy

Management

Labour cannot be stopped at this stage, but management should be aimed at delaying the delivery, if the CTG is normal, sufficient to optimize the condition of the fetus.

- *Prevention of respiratory distress syndrome (RDS)*:
  - Antenatal corticosteroids (usually intramuscular betamethasone) prior to delivery reduce the incidence of RDS in premature infants, with ideally two doses administered 12 h apart prior to delivery.
  - Tocolysis with atosiban, a beta-agonist (such as terbutaline) or nifedipine should be started immediately to try and delay labour in order for the steroids to be maximally effective (24 h), and then discontinued. The other indication for tocolysis is to settle contractions long enough for *in utero* transfer of the mother to a unit with facilities to care for a 31-week baby. In other situations tocolysis does not seem to improve fetal outcome, even though it may prolong time to delivery.
- *Magnesium sulphate*:
  - Consider intravenous magnesium sulphate for neuroprotection of the baby for women between 24+0 and 33+6 weeks of pregnancy in established preterm labour or having a planned preterm birth within 24 hours. This is to prevent neonatal seizures.
  - A 4 g intravenous bolus of magnesium sulphate is given over 15 minutes, followed by an intravenous infusion of 1 g per hour until the birth or for 24 hours (whichever is sooner).
- *Mode of delivery*: Although there is evidence that full-term singleton breech babies should be delivered by caesarean section (rather than vaginally), there is no clear evidence that

this applies to preterm infants, and as premature delivery is generally reasonably quick, vaginal delivery should be considered. The contraindications to this would be signs of fetal compromise on CTG, or maternal objection.

- *Intrapartum care*: The paediatric team should be informed of any woman in actual or threatened preterm labour, in order that appropriate arrangements are made for care of the infant after delivery.
- *Next pregnancy*: This woman should be referred to a specialist preterm birth clinic in any subsequent pregnancies where she should have serial cervical length measurements carried out by ultrasound in the second trimester, and discussion of a cervical cerclage to reduce the chance of a further preterm birth.

 KEY POINTS

- Premature delivery is the major cause of perinatal mortality.
- If a woman goes into premature labour one must consider prevention of respiratory distress syndrome, neuroprotection and mode of delivery.

CASE 84: DELIVERY

History

You are urgently called to the delivery room of a 26-year-old woman to help deliver the baby. The mother is 41 weeks into her second pregnancy, having had a normal term delivery of a 3.97 kg female infant 2 years ago.

Nuchal and anomaly scans in this pregnancy were normal and antenatal care was unremarkable. The baby was moving normally prior to labour.

When she arrived on labour ward contracting, the symphysiofundal height was noted to be 41 cm.

At first assessment the cervix was 3 cm dilated and she was advised to continue mobilizing. Spontaneous rupture of membranes occurred and she was examined again after 4 h and the cervix was still 3 cm. A syntocinon infusion was commenced to augment labour and an epidural sited, with cardiotocograph monitoring also commenced. After a further 4 h, the cervix was 7 cm and then 10 cm after another 4 h. The woman was encouraged to start active pushing and 35 min later the head had crowned in a direct occipitoanterior position.

The midwife noticed that the head did not extend normally on the perineum and that the chin appeared to be wedged against the perineum. She had attempted delivery of the shoulders with the next two contractions but this had not been achieved.

?	QUESTIONS

- What is the diagnosis?
- How would you manage this scenario?

ANSWER 84

This condition, where the fetal shoulders and trunk fail to deliver after the head, is shoulder dystocia. Complications include perinatal mortality, hypoxic encephalopathy, brachial plexus injury (e.g. Erb's palsy), as well as maternal postpartum haemorrhage and third- or fourth-degree tear.

Shoulder dystocia occurs in 1 in 200 deliveries and is associated with various risk factors (though 70 per cent of cases occur in women with no risk factors). In this case the woman had a relatively large previous baby, this baby had persistently been large on examination, she is post dates, progress was slow for a parous woman and she had required syntocinon.

!   **RISK FACTORS FOR SHOULDER DYSTOCIA**

- Estimated fetal weight (>4.5 kg)
- High BMI
- Previous big baby (>4 kg)
- Induction of labour
- South Asian ethnicity
- Gestational diabetes
- Previous shoulder dystocia
- Slow progress in the first and/or second stage of labour
- Post dates delivery
- Instrumental delivery

Management

This is an obstetric emergency and the emergency bell should be activated with help summoned from the senior midwife, other available midwives, anaesthetist and paediatrician, as well as the most senior obstetrician available.

A series of manoeuvres are practiced by labour ward staff at 'skills and drills' sessions in preparation for such an event. The first four points should be carried out in that order. If the shoulders do not then deliver, then points 5–7 can be attempted in any order, depending on the operator's experience.

1. *Call for help.*
2. *Move the patient to the end of the bed and flatten the head of the bed.*
3. *Consider episiotomy*: This will not allow the shoulders to deliver but will allow manipulation of the baby to achieve delivery.
4. *Elevate the legs* (McRoberts manoeuvre): The procedure involves flexing the maternal hips, thus positioning the thighs up onto the abdomen. This simulates the squatting position, with the advantage of increasing the inlet diameter.
5. *Suprapubic pressure*: External manual suprapubic pressure is applied to the fetus's anterior shoulder, in such a way that the shoulder will adduct or collapse anteriorly and encourage the baby's shoulder to pass under the symphysis pubis. Pressure is at first constant, and then in a rocking fashion if the baby remains undelivered.
6. *The operator's fingers should enter the pelvis*: The index and middle fingers should be inserted past the fetal head and behind the anterior shoulder, then pressure exerted on the back of that shoulder to attempt to rotate the baby (Rubin's manoeuvre). This can also be tried with the posterior shoulder from the front of the fetus, rotating the shoulder

towards the symphysis in the same direction as with the Rubin II manoeuvre (Wood screw manoeuvre).

7. *Removal of the posterior arm*: The clinician must insert his or her hand far into the vagina and locate the posterior arm. Once the arm is located, the elbow should be flexed so that the forearm may be delivered in a sweeping motion over the anterior chest wall of the fetus.

8. *Roll onto all-fours position*: If the above manoeuvres fail, the woman should be rolled onto the all-fours position which increases the true obstetrical conjugate (shortest pelvic diameter through which the fetal head must pass during birth) by as much as 10 mm and the sagittal measurement of the pelvic outlet by up to 20 mm.

Delivery usually occurs by stage 5. If it fails then last resort measures are the procedure of replacing the fetal head into the pelvis and performing emergency caesarean section (Zavanelli manoeuvre) or performing symphysiotomy (if caesarean delivery is not an option) to enlarge the pelvic diameters.

Post-Delivery

The 3 Ds of any obstetric emergency are particularly important here:

- *Document*: It is vital to have a scribe during the emergency to take down the timings of each manoeuvre and clear documentation in these cases is important to confirm which shoulder was impacted.
- *Datix*: An incident form should be filled in to allow auditing of these cases.
- *Debrief*: This is important not only for the team involved but also for the woman and birthing partner.

 KEY POINTS

- Shoulder dystocia is an obstetric emergency and requires immediate action.
- All health professionals delivering babies must be well rehearsed with the appropriate manoeuvres used to help deliver the baby.

CASE 85: HEADACHE IN PREGNANCY

History

A 17-year-old girl is admitted to the labour ward by ambulance because of a severe headache and reduced fetal movements. This is her first pregnancy. She did not discover she was pregnant until very late and was uncertain of her last menstrual period date. The pregnancy was therefore dated by ultrasound scan at 23 weeks. According to that scan she is now 37 weeks.

When she was first booked in the antenatal clinic her blood pressure was 120/68 mmHg and urinalysis negative. The blood pressure was last checked one week ago and was 132/74 mmHg and urinalysis was negative again. Booking blood tests were all normal.

This morning she woke with a frontal headache which has persisted despite paracetamol. She says that her vision is a bit blurred but she cannot be more specific about this. She also reports nausea and epigastric discomfort, but has not vomited. She denies leg or finger swelling.

Examination

The blood pressure is 164/106 mmHg. This is repeated twice at 15-min intervals and is found to be 160/110 mmHg and 164/112 mmHg. She is apyrexial and her heart rate is 83/min. Her face is minimally swollen and fundoscopy is normal. Cardiac and respiratory examinations are normal. Abdominally she is tender in the epigastrium and beneath the right costal margin, but the uterus is soft and non-tender. The fetus is cephalic and 3/5 palpable. The woman's legs and fingers are mildly oedematous and lower limb reflexes are very brisk, with clonus.

🔍 INVESTIGATIONS

		Normal Range for Pregnancy
Haemoglobin	116 g/L	110–140 g/L
Packed cell volume	42.2%	31–38%
Mean cell volume	79 fL	74.4–95.6 fL
White cell count	5×10^9/L	$6–16 \times 10^9$/L
Platelets	126×10^9/L	$150–400 \times 10^9$/L
Sodium	141 mmol/L	130–140 mmol/L
Potassium	4.0 mmol/L	3.3–4.1 mmol/L
Urea	3.8 mmol/L	2.4–4.3 mmol/L
Creatinine	92 mmol/L	34–82 mmol/L
Alanine transaminase	189 IU/L	6–32 IU/L
Alkaline phosphatase	74 IU/L	30–300 IU/L
Gamma glutamyl transaminase	34 IU/L	5–43 IU/L
Bilirubin	12 mmol/L	3–14 mmol/L
Albumin	24 g/L	28–37 g/L
Urate	0.46 mmol/L	0.14–0.38 mmol/L

Urinalysis: Protein ++++
Cardiotocograph (CTG): Baseline 140/min, reduced variability (5–10/min). Variable decelerations, occasional accelerations.

❓ QUESTIONS

- What is the diagnosis?
- How would you manage this patient?

DOI: 10.1201/9781003386933-90

ANSWER 85

The woman has pre-eclampsia with rapid onset and severity of symptoms and signs suggesting severe or 'fulminant' disease. She is at high risk of developing eclampsia.

The headache and visual disturbance are typical features of cerebral oedema; the right upper quadrant pain of subcapsular liver swelling and the proteinuria occurs from renal involvement.

The blood tests show typical features of severe pre-eclampsia:

- Elevated liver transaminases
- Elevated urate
- Elevated creatinine

The platelet count is at the lower end of the normal range for pregnancy and if reduced further, with raised bilirubin would suggest development of HELLP syndrome (haemolysis, elevated liver enzymes and low platelets).

Management

This is an obstetric emergency and the senior midwife, anaesthetist and senior obstetrician should be informed immediately. The appropriate definitive treatment for pre-eclampsia is delivery of the baby, but the maternal status must be stabilized first. In this case she should be admitted and have an intravenous cannula inserted. Blood should be sent for coagulation screen and for group and save. A urinary catheter should be inserted and fluid input and output carefully monitored for oliguria as a sign of impending renal failure.

In pre-eclampsia, although the extracellular ('third-space') fluid volume is increased, the intravascular volume is generally depleted, so fluid input should be managed carefully with the help of an anaesthetist, balancing adequate renal perfusion with the risk of overload and pulmonary oedema. Where the urine output is decreased, a central venous line may be needed for more accurate assessment of volume status.

The woman should be given an antihypertensive to reduce her blood pressure (thus reducing the risk of cerebral haemorrhage). If initial oral antihypertensives are not effective, a titrated intravenous infusion should be used.

Magnesium sulphate infusion reduces the risk of an eclamptic fit in women with severe pre-eclampsia and should be commenced immediately and continued for 24 hours post-delivery.

The CTG is found to show reduced variability and occasional variable decelerations. This suggests that the reduced fetal movements may be due to fetal distress, probably from uteroplacental insufficiency. Caesarean section would therefore be the mode of delivery of choice, but only when the maternal blood pressure is under control and the coagulation screen result is available.

Postnatally the condition may not improve for 48 h or more, and the woman should be cared for in a high-dependency setting until the blood pressure is under control, renal output is normal, symptoms have settled and blood results are returning to normal.

🔑 **KEY POINTS**

- Pre-eclampsia causes widespread endothelial dysfunction, with effects on all of the body systems. Death can occur from cerebral haemorrhage, eclampsia, pulmonary oedema, renal failure or hepatic rupture.
- Immediate stabilization of the mother should precede delivery of the baby.

History

A 36-year-old nulliparous woman at term started having uterine tightenings yesterday morning. These were intermittent initially and she managed to cope with a hot bath and paracetamol, but they have now become increasingly painful and frequent. This morning she came in because she had ruptured membranes at home an hour and a half ago. She has continued to notice normal fetal movements.

Since arrival the blood pressure, temperature and heart rate have been within the normal range and the liquor has remained clear. She has been examined several times and the findings of each examination are shown in Table 86.1. After the examination at 14.15 an oxytocin infusion was commenced.

Table 86.1 **Examination Findings**

Time	Contractions	Cervical Dilatation	Head Descent Relative to the Ischial Spines	Position	Caput	Moulding
10.30	3 in 10	3 cm	−3 cm	Left occipitotransverse	+	Nil
14.15	2 in 10	4 cm	−2 cm	Left occipitotransverse	++	Nil
Oxytocin infusion commenced						
18.20	3–4 in 10	5 cm	−2 cm	Occipitoposterior	++	+
22.15	4 in 10	6 cm	−2 cm	Occipitoposterior	+++	++

🔎 **INVESTIGATIONS**

The cardiotocograph (CTG) is shown in Figure 86.1.

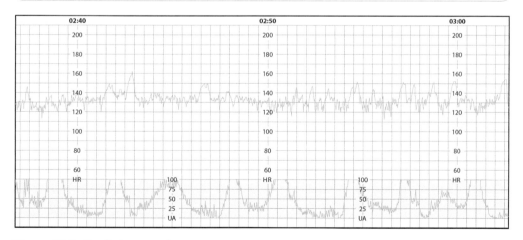

Figure 86.1 Cardiotocograph.

❓ QUESTIONS

- How do you interpret the examination and CTG findings?
- What factors are associated with this pattern of labour?
- How would you manage this woman?

DOI: 10.1201/9781003386933-91

ANSWER 86

The examination findings show failure to progress in the first stage in labour. Once labour has been established, the cervix is expected to dilate at approximately 0.5 cm/hr (1 cm/hr in women who have had a previous vaginal birth). In this case, despite attempted augmentation with an oxytocic agent, there has only been 3 cm dilatation in almost 12 h.

This situation is most common in nulliparous women and is termed primary dysfunctional labour. Other associations are malposition (commonly the occipitoposterior position) and increased fetal size (cephalopelvic disproportion).

Management

Maximum contractions have been achieved (four in 10 min) with the oxytocic for several hours, and there are increasing signs of obstruction (caput and moulding of the fetal head). In view of this the recommended management option is to perform an emergency caesarean section.

The CTG is normal, but without intervention, the likely scenario is for fetal compromise to occur. Therefore once the decision has been made to proceed with caesarean section, oxytocin should be discontinued to reduce the effect of the prolonged contractions on the baby. Delivery should be arranged within 60 min of the decision being made.

The important points in arranging delivery by emergency caesarean section in this case are:

- Informed consent, after appropriate explanation
- Informing the anaesthetist and assistant
- Informing the theatre staff and paediatrician
- Omeprazole and metoclopramide to the mother to minimize gastric aspiration should general anaesthetic be needed
- Insertion of an indwelling urinary catheter
- Transfer of the woman to theatre, with continuous CTG until delivery

---

🔑 **KEY POINTS**

- In a primigravid woman the rate of cervical dilatation in normal labour is 0.5 cm/h.
- Inefficient uterine action must be corrected with oxytocin augmentation before a diagnosis of 'failure to progress' is made.

CASE 87: POSTPARTUM BLEEDING

History

A 39-year-old woman in her first pregnancy delivered twin sons 2 h ago. There were no significant antenatal complications. She had been prescribed ferrous sulphate and folic acid during the pregnancy as anaemia prophylaxis, and her last haemoglobin was 109 g/L at 38 weeks.

The fetuses were within normal range for growth and liquor volume on serial scan estimations. A vaginal delivery was planned and she went into spontaneous labour at 37 weeks. Due to decelerations in the cardiotocograph (CTG) for the first twin, both babies were delivered by ventouse after 30 min active pushing in the second stage. The midwife recorded both placentae as appearing complete.

As this was a twin pregnancy, an intravenous cannula had been inserted when labour was established and an epidural had been sited. The lochia has been heavy since delivery but the woman is now bleeding very heavily and passing large clots of blood.

On arrival in the room you find that the sheets are soaked with blood and there is also approximately 500 mL of blood clot in a kidney dish on the bed.

Examination

The woman is conscious but drowsy and pale. The temperature is 35.9 degrees, blood pressure 120/70 mmHg and heart rate 112/min. The peripheries feel cool. The uterus is palpable to the umbilicus and feels soft. The abdomen is otherwise soft and non-tender. On vaginal inspection there is a second-degree tear which has been sutured but you are unable to assess further for soft tissue trauma due to the presence of profuse bleeding.

The midwife sent blood tests 30 min ago because she was concerned about the blood loss at the time.

🔍 INVESTIGATIONS

		Normal Range for Pregnancy
Haemoglobin	72 g/L	110–140 g/L
Mean cell volume	99.0 fL	74.4–95.6 fL
White cell count	3.2×10^9/L	$6–16 \times 10^9$/L
Platelets	131×10^9/L	$150–400 \times 10^9$/L
International normalized ratio (INR)	1.3	0.9–1.2
Activated partial thromboplastin time (APTT)	39 s	30–45 s
Sodium	138 mmol/L	130–140 mmol/L
Potassium	3.5 mmol/L	3.3–4.1 mmol/L
Urea	5.2 mmol/L	2.4–4.3 mmol/L
Creatinine	64 mmol/L	34–82 mmol/L

? QUESTIONS

- What is the diagnosis and what are the likely causes?
- What is the sequence of management options you would employ in this situation?

DOI: 10.1201/9781003386933-92

ANSWER 87

The diagnosis is primary postpartum haemorrhage (PPH), defined as the loss of more than 500 mL of blood in the first 24 h following delivery. This classification applies even if the blood is lost at caesarean section or while awaiting placental delivery.

> **! CAUSES OF AND RISK FACTORS FOR POSTPARTUM HAEMORRHAGE**
>
> - Uterine atony (multiple pregnancy, grand multiparity, polyhydramnios, prolonged labour)
> - Antepartum haemorrhage
> - Uterine sepsis (chorioamnionitis)
> - Retained placenta
> - Lower genital tract trauma (perineal or cervical tears)
> - Coagulopathy (heparin treatment, inherited or acquired bleeding disorders)
> - Previous PPH

This woman's major risk factor for bleeding is multiple pregnancy and with the high uterus, the cause is likely to be uterine atony (inability of the uterus to contract adequately). Blood loss is often underestimated, the 'high' uterus may contain a large volume of concealed blood and the blood pressure in young fit women remains relatively normal until decompensation occurs. Blood loss volume should be considered in the context of the estimated circulating blood volume of the patient (smaller women will tolerate lower volume of blood loss). In this case, the woman should be considered to be extremely sick and at risk of cardiac arrest if immediate management is not employed.

The sequence of management strategies is:

- Bimanually compress the uterus (with one hand abdominally compressing and the other hand compressing from the vagina) to expel any clots and stimulate the uterus to contract.
- Ensure two large-bore cannulae are inserted with crossmatched blood requested.
- Recheck full blood count and coagulation.
- Commence intravenous fluids for volume expansion along with O negative or type specific blood if she becomes more unstable.
- Give 500 mg ergometrine intramuscularly or intravenously to enhance uterine contraction.
- Give 1 g tranexamic acid IV.
- Start an oxytocin infusion to maintain uterine contraction.
- Consider other uterotonics such as misoprostol or carboprost (an analogue of prostaglandin F2 alpha).
- Transfer to theatre for examination under anaesthetic to assess for vaginal trauma, cervical laceration or retained placental tissue.
- The doctor or midwife should continue bimanual compression until the clinical situation is under control.
- An inflatable intrauterine balloon (Bakri balloon) should be inserted once traumatic causes of bleeding have been excluded and if uterotonics are not rapidly effective.
- If the bleeding does not settle with the above measures, and with correction of any coagulopathy, then further options are uterine artery embolization or laparotomy with B-Lynch haemostatic suture, uterine artery ligation or hysterectomy.

KEY POINTS

- Uterine compression from the abdomen or bimanually is the first and immediate management strategy for postpartum haemorrhage and should be continued until the clinical situation has settled.
- Clinicians usually underestimate blood loss and in assessing haemodynamic status may forget to take account of concealed loss (into the uterus) and the ability of healthy women to compensate.

CASE 88: LABOUR

History

A 32-year-old woman presents to the labour ward with abdominal pain. This is her first baby after two miscarriages. She was trying to conceive for 18 months prior to this pregnancy.

Her estimated delivery date was corrected after her 11–14-week scan to make her now 40 weeks and 6 days. All pregnancy blood tests and ultrasound scans have been normal. The baby was breech at 34 weeks but cephalic at 37 weeks.

This morning she had a mucus-like dark red discharge followed by the onset of irregular period-type pains. Two hours ago she felt a gush of clear fluid from the vagina and since then the pains have become much more severe, now occurring every 4 min, lasting for 45 s.

The baby has moved normally during the day.

She had a bath at home and took paracetamol but is now distressed and has come to hospital for assessment. Her partner and sister who are both very anxious accompany her.

Examination

On examination she is comfortable between pains. Her blood pressure is 129/76 mmHg and pulse 101/min. Symphysiofundal height is 37 cm and the fetus is cephalic with 2/5 palpable.

Speculum examination shows clear fluid pooled in the posterior vaginal fornix.

Vaginal examination reveals the cervix to be fully effaced and 4 cm dilated. The position is right occipitoposterior and the head is 2 cm above the ischial spines. There is no fetal caput or moulding.

🔍 INVESTIGATIONS

Urinalysis: Blood ++
Proteinuria: +
Leucocytes: Negative
Nitrites: Negative

? QUESTIONS

- What is the diagnosis?
- What is the appropriate management?

DOI: 10.1201/9781003386933-93

ANSWER 88

This woman is in normal labour.

> ! **DEFINITION OF LABOUR**
>
> The onset of regular painful contractions with progressive dilatation of the cervix and descent of the presenting part.

Spontaneous rupture of membranes has occurred in this case but is not necessary for the diagnosis of labour.

The woman's observations and examination findings are normal for labour:

- The dark mucus discharge is a 'show' and is not a cause for concern unless the bleeding is fresh or ongoing.
- The pulse is almost certainly raised secondarily to the pain.
- The haematuria and proteinuria are secondary to contamination by the show and liquor.
- The symphysiofundal height is low because the head has descended into the pelvis and because the liquor has been released from the uterus.

Management

The pregnancy and labour are low risk in that there is no evidence of any fetal or maternal disorder that requires doctor-led care. The woman should therefore remain under midwife-led care and does not need continuous electronic fetal monitoring (cardiotocograph [CTG]). The fetus does however need assessment for wellbeing with intermittent auscultation for a full minute after a contraction at least every 15 min in the first stage of labour and for a full minute after a contraction every 5 min in the second stage of labour.

The progress of the labour should be recorded on a partogram, which should include maternal and fetal observations.

> ! **MONITORING IN LOW-RISK LABOUR**
>
> - Hourly blood pressure
> - Hourly heart rate
> - Four-hourly examinations for cervical dilatation
> - Assessment for meconium

Once labour is established, expected dilatation is approximately 0.5 cm/h. If this does not occur or if signs suggest that fetal or maternal wellbeing might be compromised, then medical assessment and possible intervention may be indicated.

> 🔑 **KEY POINTS**
>
> - Normal labour is the onset of regular painful contractions with progressive dilatation of the cervix and descent of the presenting part.
> - Continuous CTG is not required for low-risk women in normal labour, but intermittent auscultation is essential.

CASE 89: PAIN IN PREGNANCY

History

A 35-year-old woman arrives on the labour ward complaining of abdominal pain and vaginal bleeding at 36 weeks 2 days' gestation. The pain started 2 h earlier while she was in a café. She describes constant pain all over her abdomen with exacerbations every few minutes. It is not relieved by lying still or by walking around. The vaginal bleeding is bright red and was initially noticed on the toilet paper but now has stained her underclothes and trousers. There are no urinary or bowel symptoms.

The baby has been moving normally until today, but the woman has not paid any attention to the movements since the pain started.

This is her first pregnancy and until now progress has been uneventful with shared care between the general practitioner and midwife. Both the 11–14-week and the anomaly scan at 20 weeks were reassuring. Booking and subsequent blood test results were normal. The booking blood pressure was 112/68 mmHg and the most recent blood pressure 2 days ago was 128/80 mmHg.

Examination

She is obviously in significant pain and feels clammy. She is apyrexial, her heart rate is 115/min and blood pressure 110/62 mmHg. The symphysiofundal height is 38 cm and the uterus feels hard and is very tender. It is not possible to feel the presentation of the fetus due to the uterine tightening. On speculum examination there is a trickle of blood through the cervix and the cervix appears closed. Vaginal examination reveals that the cervix is soft and almost fully effaced but closed. No fetal heart sounds are heard on auscultation with the hand-held fetal Doppler. Ultrasound scan confirms that the fetus has died.

INVESTIGATIONS

		Normal Range for Pregnancy
Haemoglobin	81 g/L	110–140 g/L
White cell count	6×10^9/L	6–16×10^9/L
Platelets	93×10^9/L	150–400×10^9/L
Sodium	137 mmol/L	130–140 mmol/L
Potassium	4.0 mmol/L	3.3–4.1 mmol/L
Urea	6.5 mmol/L	2.4–4.3 mmol/L
Creatinine	82 mmol/L	34–82 mmol/L
International normalized ratio (INR)	2.2	0.9–1.2
Activated partial thromboplastin time (APTT)	34 s	30–45 s

QUESTIONS

- What is the diagnosis?
- How do you interpret the examination and blood test findings?
- How would you manage this patient?

DOI: 10.1201/9781003386933-94

ANSWER 89

The pain and bleeding are due to placental abruption. In this case the presence of vaginal blood classifies it as a 'revealed abruption' but the other signs of a hardened 'couvelaire' uterus, raised symphysiofundal height, tachycardia and low haemoglobin all suggest that the majority of the blood volume lost is still 'concealed'. This is an extremely important point as the amount of visualized blood can be misleading when there may be 1–2 L of blood concealed within the uterus.

The blood pressure appears normal, but this is because the woman is relatively young and fit – she is able to compensate for the blood loss by increasing her heart rate and cardiac output for some time. By the time her blood pressure falls she has decompensated and is critically unwell, so one should not be falsely reassured by normal blood pressure in young people. If her blood pressure were checked lying and standing, there would be a significant difference, which would reveal the extent of her hypovolaemia.

The increase in INR and decreased platelets confirm that the woman has developed disseminated intravascular coagulopathy (DIC) as a result of the abruption.

The fetus has died (intrauterine fetal death) because the placenta has separated from the uterus and the uteroplacental circulation has therefore been interrupted.

Management

This is an obstetric emergency as the woman is hypovolaemic and has developed a coagulopathy. The management should be focused on correction of the clotting derangement and volume replacement as well as delivery of the baby. A senior anaesthetist and senior obstetrician should liaise closely in management. The haematology team should also be alerted as the need for a significant amount of packed red cells and clotting factors should be anticipated.

!　RESUSCITATION OF THE MOTHER (INITIAL BASIC PROCEDURES)

- Insertion of two large-bore venous cannulae.
- Request urgent crossmatch of 6 units of blood.
- Request fresh-frozen plasma and platelets.
- Initial fluid resuscitation with intravenous fluids +/– blood products.
- Insertion of a urinary catheter to monitor urine output.

Even though the baby has died, a caesarean section may be indicated to aid with resuscitation of the mother. If the woman was already in established labour then this could be expedited if necessary with oxytocin infusion and would usually progress quickly, though the woman would need very close monitoring for signs of compromise. Postpartum haemorrhage is common after an abruption and steps should be taken to minimise this.

　KEY POINTS

- Placental abruption is an obstetric emergency and must be aggressively managed as disseminated intravascular coagulation can develop rapidly.
- Placental abruption is commonly associated with the development of pre-eclampsia.
- Labour can progress rapidly, however caesarean section may still be needed even in the context of an intrauterine death to stabilize the woman.
- Postpartum haemorrhage is very likely after an abruption.

History

A woman has just delivered her second baby on the labour ward. She is 37 years old and had a previous premature delivery at 34 weeks. In this pregnancy she went into spontaneous labour at 38 weeks after an uncomplicated pregnancy.

The symphysiofundal height was consistent with dates until 37 weeks when the midwife measured it as 41 cm. However before an ultrasound scan for growth and liquor volume could be arranged the woman went into spontaneous labour.

At the time of admission with contractions she was 5 cm dilated and spontaneous rupture of membranes occurred soon after. The baby was delivered 30 min later in the direct occipitoanterior position.

The placenta was delivered by controlled cord traction, and the midwife confirmed that the uterus was well contracted following this, with an estimated total blood loss during delivery of approximately 250 mL. However on examination of the perineum they noticed a perineal tear. The tear extended from the introitus posteriorly in the midline and the midwife could see torn muscle fibres suggestive of the torn ends of the external anal sphincter. She has called you to review the patient.

? | **QUESTIONS**

- What is the likely diagnosis?
- What factors predispose to this condition?
- How would you manage this patient?

DOI: 10.1201/9781003386933-95

ANSWER 90

The history suggests a third-degree tear.

> **!** | **CLASSIFICATION OF PERINEAL TEARS**
>
> - *First degree*: Injury to the perineum involving the epithelium or skin but not the perineal muscles
> - *Second degree*: Injury to the perineum involving perineal muscles but not involving the anal sphincter
> - *Third degree*: Injury to the perineum involving the anal sphincter complex (external anal sphincter [EAS] and internal anal sphincter [IAS]):
>   - 3a: Less than 50 per cent of EAS thickness torn
>   - 3b: More than 50 per cent of EAS thickness torn
>   - 3c: IAS torn
> - *Fourth degree*: Injury to the perineum involving the anal sphincter complex (EAS and IAS) and rectal mucosa

Risk Factors

A third-degree tear occurs in 2–4 per cent of women at delivery, and is more common in the following circumstances:

- Birth weight over 4 kg
- Persistent occipitoposterior position
- Asian ethnicity
- Nulliparity
- Induction of labour
- Second stage of labour lasting more than 1 h
- Instrumental delivery

Third-degree tear diagnosis depends on the vigilance of the person inspecting a tear and may easily be missed. This has far-reaching consequences, as failure to perform adequate primary repair may increase the chance of longer-term faecal incontinence.

Management

- The woman should be transferred to theatre for repair. This enables adequate analgesia (spinal or epidural), full lithotomy position for proper exposure of the tissues, good lighting and availability of appropriate instruments and space for an assistant if needed.
- The tear should be repaired in layers:
  - Rectal mucosa (if involved)
  - Internal anal sphincter (if involved)
  - External anal sphincter
  - Perineal muscle
  - Vaginal epithelium
  - Perineal skin
- Broad-spectrum antibiotics should be administered to prevent infection from possible contamination by bowel organisms.
- Laxatives should be administered to prevent constipation that might compromise the repair.
- Adequate postoperative analgesia is needed.

- Information should be given about pelvic floor exercises and a referral to a specialist women's health physiotherapist should be made.
- A follow-up appointment should be arranged for approximately 6 weeks after delivery to ensure that the woman has no significant bowel symptoms, to allow for anal sphincter ultrasound and to refer on to a colorectal specialist if there are ongoing concerns with continence or bowel control.
- Elective caesarean section should be discussed as a possibility for any subsequent deliveries if she has ongoing symptoms.

 KEY POINTS

- Following delivery any vaginal tear must be inspected carefully to ensure that the anal sphincter is not disrupted.
- All third-degree tears should be repaired in theatre by an experienced operator to minimise the chance of future problems with faecal incontinence.

CASE 91: FITS IN PREGNANCY

History

An obviously pregnant woman is brought to the emergency department having suffered a seizure in the park 20 min ago. She had been alone at the time but the seizure was witnessed by another woman who said that she had stood up from a bench and then suddenly dropped to the ground. She thought she may have hit her head on the side of the bench with the fall. Her arms and legs had been shaking and then were 'stiff and trembling' for about 40 s. The woman's face had gone dusky and there was some frothing at the mouth. She noticed that the woman's trousers were wet afterwards.

When the fit stopped the woman had appeared unconscious for a few minutes and then showed some response to being talked to but seemed confused and drowsy.

Examination

She appears to be about 30 years old and in the third trimester of pregnancy. She is now conscious but still drowsy and her Glasgow Coma Scale is 9/15.

Her blood pressure is 140/98 mmHg and heart rate 104/min. Examination shows no obvious cardiac or chest abnormality, and on abdominal palpation there is no apparent tenderness. The uterus feels approximately 30 weeks in size (midway between umbilicus and xiphisternum), and a fetus can be palpated, cephalic with 4/5 palpable. Reflexes are brisk and plantar reflexes are upgoing.

INVESTIGATIONS

No investigation results are yet available for this patient when you see her.

? QUESTIONS

- What is your provisional diagnosis and how would you manage this woman in the first instance?
- The woman's husband arrives shortly and explains that she is a known epileptic who has grand mal seizures every few days, despite drug treatment. How should your management alter now?

DOI: 10.1201/9781003386933-96

ANSWER 91

Any woman with a fit in the second half of pregnancy should be assumed to have eclampsia until proven otherwise. The risks of maternal or perinatal mortality are so great that it is better to treat the woman for eclampsia and prevent a further seizure than to spend time investigating and making a certain diagnosis while risking further fits. This case is therefore an obstetric emergency (despite the fact that the fit resolved spontaneously), and help should be summoned from the anaesthetist, senior midwife, senior obstetrician and paediatrician.

Magnesium sulphate should be given as an intravenous bolus of 4 g, followed by an infusion in normal saline of 1 g/h (increased if further fits occur).

Once this has been commenced, the blood pressure should be checked, with intravenous antihypertensives started if appropriate. A urine sample should be acquired (with insertion of a Foley catheter to monitor urine output) for proteinuria. Fluid input should be restricted initially to 85 mL/h. Blood should be sent for full blood count, urea and electrolytes, urate, liver function tests, coagulation screen and group and save. She should be transferred to a high-dependency area of the labour ward with continuous electrocardiogram and cardiotocograph monitoring.

Once stable and when further investigations have been made into her previous history, a decision can be made regarding delivery.

Epilepsy Diagnosis

The fact that the woman has epilepsy strongly suggests that this fit is caused by the epilepsy. However the initial management was still correct as it should not be assumed that the fit was due to epilepsy until the urinalysis has been confirmed to be normal and the blood pressure, initially high, has normalized and the blood tests results are confirmed to be normal.

Reflexes are commonly brisk in the postictal phase, with upgoing plantar responses. The reflexes would be expected to return to normal if the seizure was due to epilepsy but not if the diagnosis was of eclampsia.

This woman regained full consciousness after half an hour and the blood pressure was normal with negative urinalysis and normal blood results. The magnesium was thus discontinued and she was reviewed by the neurological team with adjustments made to her regular epilepsy medication.

 KEY POINT

- A woman who presents in the third trimester of pregnancy with a grand mal seizure should be treated as eclamptic until proven otherwise.

CASE 92: BREATHLESSNESS IN PREGNANCY

History

A 42-year-old woman is referred by her general practitioner with breathlessness for the past 3 days. She is 34 weeks pregnant in her third pregnancy. Prior to the current pregnancy she had an emergency caesarean section for abnormal cardiotocograph in labour at term, followed by a 7-week miscarriage.

In this pregnancy she was seen by the obstetric consultant to discuss plans for delivery, and is hoping for a vaginal delivery. Ultrasound scans and blood tests have been normal. Her booking blood pressure was 138/80 mmHg and has remained stable during the pregnancy.

She describes her shortness of breath starting while she was at work and slightly worsening since. She felt particularly breathless when she ran to catch a bus on her way home yesterday. She has some left-sided chest pain on breathing in. There is no cough or haemoptysis. She has had no previous episodes. She has not noticed any calf pain but has left leg swelling and some back pain.

Examination

The BMI is 28 kg/m^2. The woman does not look obviously unwell. Blood pressure is 127/78 mmHg and heart rate 98/min. Oxygen saturation is 96 per cent on air. On examination of the chest there is a systolic murmur and no added sounds. Chest expansion is normal but the woman reports pain on taking a deep breath. The chest is resonant to percussion and chest sounds are normal except for a pleural rub on the left. The left leg is generally swollen but no redness or tenderness is apparent.

🔍 INVESTIGATIONS

		Normal Range for Pregnancy
Haemoglobin	120 g/L	110–140 g/L
White cell count	10.4×10^9/L	$6–16 \times 10^9$/L
Platelets	302×10^9/L	346×10^9/L
Arterial blood gas (on air)		
PaO$_2$	11.0 kPa	12–14 kPa
PaCO$_2$	5.3 kPa	5–6 kPa

- Electrocardiogram (ECG): Sinus tachycardia 100/min, deep S wave in lead 1, Q wave in lead 3 and inverted T wave in lead 3.
- Chest X-ray: Normal.

Computerized tomography pulmonary angiogram (CTPA) is shown in Figure 92.1.

DOI: 10.1201/9781003386933-97

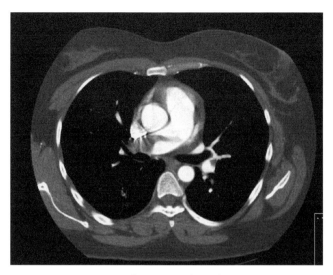

Figure 92.1 Computed tomography pulmonary angiogram.

- What is the diagnosis?
- What further imaging is required?
- How would you manage this woman in the immediate term, during delivery and postnatally?

ANSWER 92

The diagnosis is of pulmonary embolism (PE). The shortness of breath and pleuritic chest pain are classic features, and the ECG and blood gas analysis support the diagnosis. The CTPA demonstrates a large filling defect within the right pulmonary artery and a smaller filling defect in the left segmental pulmonary artery, consistent with blood clots (pulmonary embolism). These findings are illustrated by the arrows in Figure 92.2.

Venous thromboembolism (VTE) is a leading cause of direct deaths in the Confidential Enquiry into Maternal and Child Health, accounting for death in 1 per 100,000 maternities. Non-fatal VTE occurs in approximately 60 in 10,000 pregnancies, and there may be many more unrecognized cases. Pregnancy itself is a risk factor because of the hyperoestrogenic state, the altered blood viscosity and obstruction to venous blood flow by the gravid uterus.

Further Imaging

Leg swelling and back pain are suspicious of an ileofemoral deep vein thrombosis, even in the absence of skin redness. If this is confirmed, which may require Doppler ultrasound or magnetic resonance imaging (or if she develops recurrent PE despite anticoagulation), then liaison with a vascular team should be considered regarding the possibility of insertion of a vena caval filter.

Management

As with non-pregnant patients, anticoagulation is the mainstay of treatment. Warfarin is contraindicated in the first trimester of pregnancy but may safely be given from 12 to 36 weeks. However it can cause difficulties with excessive bleeding if it is not stopped early enough before delivery and it can be difficult to achieve stable international normalized ratio levels. Therefore low-molecular-weight heparin has become the treatment of choice in pregnancy as it is simple to administer, relatively easy to reverse in the emergency situation, does not require monitoring and is safe.

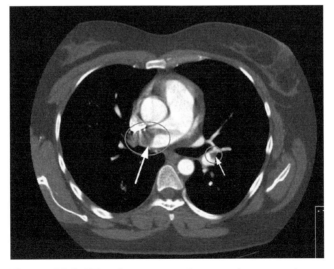

Figure 92.2 CT pulmonary angiogram demonstrating a large filling defect in the right main pulmonary artery (large arrow) and smaller defect in a segmental branch of the left pulmonary artery (smaller arrow).

At delivery the heparin should ideally be discontinued 12 h before delivery and recommenced immediately following delivery. Similarly an epidural or spinal anaesthetic should not be administered within 12 hours after a heparin dose.

Postnatally some women change to warfarin, which is now known to be safe with breast-feeding, while others continue low-molecular-weight heparin.

A large proportion of VTE occurs postnatally, so anticoagulation should be continued for 6 weeks to 3 months in the puerperium.

Graduated elastic compression stockings should be worn from the time of diagnosis until at least 6 weeks following delivery, to reduce the risk of the postthrombotic syndrome (chronic leg pain, swelling and ulceration).

Postnatal investigation for inherited (e.g. protein C or S deficiency) or acquired (e.g. antiphospholipid syndrome) thrombophilia is appropriate, as is anticoagulation throughout any subsequent pregnancy.

KEY POINTS

- Thromboembolic disease is common in pregnancy and one should have a high index of suspicion in making the diagnosis clinically.
- Often women will present with only subtle signs such as tachycardia so a low threshold for investigation is important.
- Therapeutic dose anticoagulation should be given immediately on suspicion of venous thromboembolism while waiting for confirmation of the diagnosis.

CASE 93: BLOOD PRESSURE AND PREGNANCY

History

A woman was admitted from the antenatal clinic 2 days ago at 38 weeks' gestation. She is 42 years old and this is her second pregnancy. Her first child was born by spontaneous vaginal delivery 13 years ago. She has subsequently remarried. Her booking blood pressure was 138/70 mmHg at 13 weeks. Her booking blood tests were unremarkable. At her 36-week midwife appointment 2 weeks ago, her blood pressure was 140/85 mmHg and the urinalysis was normal. The blood pressure was repeated 2 days later and was 140/82 mmHg. Two days ago she saw her midwife for a further appointment and her blood pressure was 148/101 mmHg. Urinalysis showed protein +.

She feels well in herself except for swollen legs. She denies any headache or blurring of vision.

Examination

She has oedema to the midcalves and her fingers are swollen such that she cannot remove her rings. Abdominal palpation is non-tender and the symphysiofundal height is 39 cm. Reflexes are normal.

🔍 INVESTIGATIONS

		Normal Range for Pregnancy
Haemoglobin	124 g/L	110–140 g/L
White cell count	8×10^9/L	6–16×10^9/L
Packed cell volume	34%	31–38%
Platelets	210×10^9/L	150–400×10^9/L
Sodium	137 mmol/L	130–140 mmol/L
Potassium	3.9 mmol/L	3.3–4.1 mmol/L
Urea	2.5 mmol/L	2.4–4.3 mmol/L
Creatinine	80 mmol/L	34–82 mmol/L
Alanine transaminase	37 IU/L	6–32 IU/L
Alkaline phosphatase	98 IU/L	30–300 IU/L
Bilirubin	10 mmol/L	(3–14 micromol/L)
Gamma glutamyl transaminase	32 IU/L	5–43 IU/L
Urate	43 mmol/L	(0.14–0.38 mmol/L)

Urine PCR 100 (<30).

❓ QUESTIONS

- How would you interpret the investigations?
- What further investigations are needed and how should she be managed?

DOI: 10.1201/9781003386933-98

ANSWER 93

Results Interpretation

The haemoglobin and packed cell volume suggest mild haemoconcentration. The platelet count is normal for pregnancy, though low for a non-pregnant person. Electrolytes are within the normal range but the creatinine is higher than normal for pregnancy. Alkaline phosphatase is always raised in pregnancy due to its production by the placenta. However, the alanine trans-aminase is abnormal.

A normal urate value correlates with gestational age (the urate level should not be more than the number of weeks gestation) and therefore the level of 43 mmol/L is high. Finally, the urinary PCR is high showing a large volume of proteinuria.

This woman thus has pregnancy-induced hypertension (PIH) with proteinuria, abnormal liver function and raised serum creatinine and urate. This is known as pre-eclampsia. The condition commonly occurs in asymptomatic women and the severity of symptoms often does not correlate with the disease severity.

No further maternal investigations are needed at this stage but fetal wellbeing needs to be assessed by cardiotocograph and ultrasound assessment for fetal growth and liquor volume in view of the association between pre-eclampsia and intrauterine growth restriction.

Induction of labour as soon as possible is indicated, as the fetus is mature (beyond 37 weeks) and delay might increase the likelihood of fulminating pre-eclampsia in the mother or fetal compromise, including placental abruption. There is no indication for caesarean section unless induction is unsuccessful or fetal compromise occurs before or during labour. Close monitoring of blood pressure is imperative during and after labour, as many eclamptic fits occur postnatally.

In this case the woman agreed to induction of labour and started contracting after the first dose of intravaginal prostaglandin gel. The labour progressed rapidly with subsequent normal delivery. However the blood pressure increased in labour to 155/110 mmHg. An epidural was sited to help reduce the blood pressure. Blood pressure increased further and a labetalol infusion was required.

She remained in hospital for 5 days postpartum for blood pressure monitoring, during which time her blood results returned to normal. Postnatally she was converted to oral labetalol for 6 weeks, after which blood pressure was normal, and treatment discontinued.

  KEY POINTS

- Pre-eclampsia is common and is associated with significant maternal morbidity and mortality.
- Proteinuria should be quantified with a urinary protein:creatinine ratio.

CASE 94: LABOUR

History

A 22-year-old woman is admitted to the labour ward for induction of labour at 40 weeks' gestation. This is her first ongoing pregnancy, having had a first-trimester miscarriage 13 months previously. She booked at 9 weeks and had normal booking blood tests. The 11–14-week scan and 21-week anomaly scan did not show any fetal abnormality. Blood pressure and urinalysis have always been normal.

At her 32-week midwife appointment she had reported feeling very uncomfortable abdominally, and the midwife measured the symphysiofundal height to be 36 cm. A further ultrasound scan was therefore requested which showed normal fetal growth but increased liquor volume. She had been reviewed in the antenatal clinic and was tested for gestational diabetes with a glucose tolerance test but this was normal. Subsequent examinations had again confirmed an increased symphysiofundal height, with further ultrasound scan at 36 weeks again showing normal growth, no fetal abnormality and markedly increased liquor volume. The fetal movements have always been normal.

A decision had been made for induction of labour at 40 weeks because the woman had become so uncomfortable and breathless.

On palpation the fetus was cephalic with the head 4/5 palpable abdominally. Cardiotocograph (CTG) was reassuring; 2 mg of prostaglandin gel had been inserted into the posterior fornix of the vagina and CTG monitoring continued for a further 20 min.

The woman then mobilized and contractions started within an hour. She requested an epidural for analgesia and while this was being prepared CTG monitoring was commenced. At this stage, spontaneous rupture of membranes occurred with a very large volume of clear liquor soaking the bed sheets.

  INVESTIGATIONS

The CTG is shown in Figure 94.1.

DOI: 10.1201/9781003386933-99

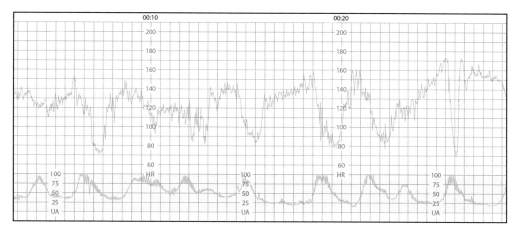

Figure 94.1 Cardiotocograph.

? QUESTIONS

- Describe the CTG.
- What is the likely diagnosis?
- How would you confirm the diagnosis and manage this situation?

ANSWER 94

The CTG shows deep atypical variable decelerations. The sudden CTG deterioration after rupture of membranes in a woman with polyhydramnios suggests the likelihood of prolapse of the cord. Other possible diagnoses are placental abruption or fetal head compression from precipitate labour. The diagnosis is easily confirmed with vaginal examination. A loop of umbilical cord will be palpated in the vagina and will be pulsatile.

! RISK FACTORS FOR CORD PROLAPSE

- Polyhydramnios
- Preterm delivery
- Malpresentation
- Unstable presentation
- Multiple pregnancy

This is an obstetric emergency and the emergency bell should be activated with the senior midwife, theatre team, senior obstetrician, paediatrician and anaesthetist summoned immediately.

The important management steps are:

- The examiner should not remove their fingers from the vagina and should attempt to elevate the fetal head to relieve pressure on the cord and minimize contact with the cord to prevent spasm.
- The woman can be rotated into the 'all-fours position' (head lower than buttocks), which will further facilitate relieving the weight of the baby and abdomen from the prolapsed cord.
- She should be transferred to theatre immediately for caesarean section.
- Intravenous access should be obtained, and a general anaesthetic administered, using a rapid sequence induction with cricoid pressure unless a very quick spinal can be achieved along with normalization of the CTG.
- The examiner should only remove their fingers from the presenting part in the vagina when the uterus has been opened and the baby is being delivered.

🔑 KEY POINTS

- Cord prolapse should be suspected in cases of fetal heart abnormality occurring after rupture of membranes.
- Cord prolapse is an obstetric emergency and necessitates immediate caesarean section.
- Attempts should be made to minimize pressure on the cord pending delivery.

Section 6

FAMILY PLANNING AND SEXUAL HEALTH

CASE 95: POSTNATAL CONTRACEPTION

History

A 36-year-old woman comes to the antenatal clinic in her third pregnancy and wants to talk about contraception options. She has had two previous spontaneous vaginal deliveries 5 and 3 years ago and has two healthy children. This was an unplanned pregnancy and she does not wish to have any further children following the forthcoming delivery.

She plans on breast-feeding this baby for at least 6 months as she did with her previous children.

The BMI is 23 kg/m^2 and she has never smoked. She has no history of VTE or any family history of breast cancer.

Her periods were regular before pregnancy and heavy for the first 2–3 days (changing protection sometimes every 2 hours). She used the combined oral contraceptive pill before her first pregnancy and did not experience any side effects.

> **?** | **QUESTIONS**
>
> • What postnatal contraceptive options are available to this woman?
> • What value is there in having this conversation during pregnancy rather than advising her to discuss contraception with her GP after the delivery?

ANSWER 95

In the UK contraception advice should follow the Medical Eligibility Criteria (UK MEC) rating system published by the Faculty of Sexual and Reproductive Health. Each personal characteristic or medical condition is given a category which indicates the safety of use of that contraceptive method as follows:

- *Category 1*: A condition for which there is no restriction for the use of method.
- *Category 2*: A condition where the advantages of using the method generally outweigh the risks.
- *Category 3*: A condition where the theoretical or proven risks usually outweigh the risk in using the method. If still wishes to use then referral to a specialist contraceptive provider is advised.
- *Category 4*: A condition which represents an unacceptable health risk if the method is used.

The guidance includes specific advice on contraception in the postnatal period.

Condition	Cu-IUD	LNG-IUS	IMP	DMPA	POP	CHC
Postpartum (in breast-feeding women)						
a) 0 to <6 weeks	See below		1	2	1	4
b) ≥6 weeks to >6 months (primarily breast-feeding)			1	1	1	3
c) ≥6 months			1	1	1	1
Postpartum (in non-breast-feeding women)						
a) 0 to <3 weeks	See below					
(i) With other risk factors for VTE*			1	2	1	4
(ii) Without other risk factors			1	2	1	3
b) 3 to <6 weeks						
(i) With other risk factors for VTE*			1	2	1	3
(ii) Without other risk factors			1	1	1	2
c) ≥6 weeks			1	1	1	1
Postpartum (in breast-feeding or non-breast-feeding women, including post-caesarean section)						
a) 0 to <48 hours	1	1	See above			
b) 48 hours to < 4 weeks	3	3				
c) >4 weeks	1	1				
d) Postpartum sepsis	4	4				

*In the presence of other risk factors for VTE, including immobility, transfusion at delivery, BMI ≥30 kg/m², postpartum haemorrhage, post-caesarean delivery, pre-eclampsia or smoking, use of CHC may pose an additional increased risk for VTE.
Source: Faculty for Sexual and Reproductive Health guideline on contraception after pregnancy (UKMEC 2016).

Breast-feeding alone should not be considered a reliable means of inhibiting ovulation and preventing pregnancy. The combined contraceptive pill is not also suitable for this woman postnatally in view of the increased thrombotic risk in the puerperium.

The progesterone-only pill is however suitable or alternatively a long acting reversible (LARC) method, such as the contraceptive implant or an intrauterine device, as the chance of missing pills is considered high in the context of caring for a new baby.

The levonorgestrel-releasing intrauterine device can be inserted immediately following delivery of the placenta, with follow-up to ensure the position is correct and to have the threads of the coil trimmed if required. Although the risk of spontaneous expulsion of the device is higher than if not inserted at the time of delivery (1 in 7 compared to 1 in 20), most women find this an acceptable risk. If it was necessary for the woman to undergo caesarean section, then the device can also be inserted (through the uterine incision) at the time. However insertion between 48 hours and 4 weeks after the delivery is not recommended as the risk of uterine perforation is considered unacceptably high.

Advantages of this form of contraception are its reliability, safety with breast-feeding and beneficial effect on reducing heavy menstrual bleeding.

If it was necessary to carry out a caesarean section then there is the added option of tubal sterilization during the procedure. This should always have been discussed and agreed to in the antenatal period as the levels of regret are high when sterilization is carried out following delivery. The failure rate of sterilization is quoted as 1 in 200 so it is not as effective as the levonorgestrel-releasing coil but it does not have any associated side effects and should be considered if the woman is sure that her family is complete.

The value of this conversation in the antenatal period is that the woman can make a plan for immediate contraception commencement at the time of or following delivery, having had time to consider and discuss the implications of each option.

 KEY POINTS

- Postnatal contraception should be discussed in the antenatal period.
- Medical eligibility criteria guidelines should be followed as for any woman requiring contraception.
- The most appropriate contraception after delivery depends on the type of delivery, whether she intends to breast-feed and how soon after delivery the woman requires protection.

CASE 96: CONTRACEPTION

History

A woman has been referred by her GP for contraceptive advice. She is 28 years old and had a thromboembolism at the age of 24 years following a triathlon event and long rail journey home. Prior to this she was using the combined oral contraceptive pill for contraception. She uses condoms reliably but has recently had an unplanned pregnancy as a result of a split condom, despite using the emergency contraception after the event. She terminated the pregnancy and feels deeply upset about the experience.

She is desperate for reliable contraception. She was advised to try the copper intrauterine contraception device but has read that this may worsen her already heavy periods. She has also discussed the progesterone-only pill with her GP but is scared that she may forget to take it at precisely the right time every day and therefore be at risk of further pregnancy.

Her cycle is regular, bleeding for 5 days every 30 days. She has had no other pregnancies and no relevant gynaecological problems. She has no other significant medical history and takes no regular medications.

She works as a marketing consultant with a fairly busy overseas travel schedule. She has been in a stable relationship with her partner for 3 years, but they do not plan to start a family in the near future.

?	QUESTION
	• What are the contraceptive options to her and their relative advantages and disadvantages?

DOI: 10.1201/9781003386933-102

ANSWER 96

Oestrogen-containing contraception is contraindicated for this woman because of her history of venous thromboembolism, even though the thrombosis in the case was apparently provoked by the situational events at the time. This means that the options are progesterone-only methods or non-hormonal methods.

Although her compliance with barrier contraception is good, she has had a distressing experience as a result of a split condom and failure of the emergency contraception, so these are probably not appropriate options for her to continue. The copper intrauterine contraceptive device would be effective in preventing pregnancy though likely to worsen her periods, as she has read, and therefore would not be a first-line choice.

The progesterone-only pill is reasonably effective (Pearl index 0.3–4/100 women-years) but this is highly correlated with compliance. In this woman's case the busy schedule and travel may mean that she is unable to reliably take the pill within the necessary 12 h time frame. Thus she may be better advised to consider a long-acting method.

Long-Acting Reversible Contraception

The five methods of long-acting reversible contraception include the copper coil, the contraceptive vaginal ring, the contraceptive implant, the contraceptive injection and the levonorgestrel-containing intrauterine system (IUS).

Copper Intrauterine Device

As described this is unlikely to be a suitable option for this woman as she already has menorrhagia which is likely to be worsened by the coil.

Contraceptive Vaginal Ring

This flexible transparent plastic ring is placed in the vagina where it releases oestrogen and progestogen. It is left *in situ* for 21 days and then removed for 7 days before a further ring is inserted. It is highly effective (Pearl index less than 1) but contraindicated in this case because of the history of thrombosis.

Levonorgestrel-Containing Intrauterine System (IUS)

The advantages are the high efficacy (Pearl index 0.2) and the fact that it can be left *in situ* for up to 3–5 years (depending on which device is used). Fertility returns within a few days following removal. Within 12 months of device insertion, many women are oligoamenorrhoeic or amenorrhoeic which is an advantage to some though disconcerting to others.

Disadvantages are that it may cause discomfort at fitting (though uterine perforation is rare) and importantly can be associated with irregular bleeding or spotting during the first 6 months of use. Although the amount of systemic levonorgestrel absorption is low, some women report progestogenic side effects of acne, low mood or bloating but again these tend to lessen over the first 6 months.

Contraceptive Implant

The contraceptive subdermal implant is a 4 cm flexible rod containing etonogestrel which is inserted into the woman's upper inner arm under local anaesthetic. It has the advantage of being highly effective (Pearl index less than 0.5) and can be left *in situ* for 3 years before replacement or removal. There is no delay in fertility after removal. The main disadvantage is the frequency (50 per cent) of bleeding irregularity which may be heavy or erratic. However unlike the contraceptive injection, the implant can be removed to resolve this. Acne can worsen with the implant but changes in mood, weight, libido and headaches are not proven side effects.

Contraceptive Injection

The contraceptive injection involves a deep intramuscular dose of depot medroxyprogesterone acetate every 12 weeks or norethisterone enanthate every 8 weeks. The advantages are the ease of administration compared with the implant or IUS and high efficacy (Pearl index less than 0.5).

Amenorrhoea is very common but many women may experience persistent irregular bleeding. There is a significant increase in weight with injectable contraceptives (up to 2–3 kg in 1 year) and a small loss in bone density (which recovers on discontinuation). In addition there may be a delayed return of fertility for up to 1 year following discontinuation.

> **!** **CONSIDERATIONS WHEN MAKING A DECISION ABOUT CONTRACEPTIVE METHODS**
>
> - Contraceptive efficacy (commonly described using the Pearl index = number of pregnancies if 100 women used this method with perfect compliance for 12 months)
> - Likely duration of use
> - Risks and side effects
> - Individual contraindications for use (e.g. previous thrombosis or migraine with aura and oestrogen contraceptives)
> - Non-contraceptive benefits (e.g. prevention of sexually transmitted infection with condoms, control of menorrhagia with combined contraceptive pill)
> - Procedure for initiation/insertion/removal
> - Possible delay in fertility after use

> **KEY POINTS**
>
> - History of venous thromboembolism is an absolute contraindication for oestrogen-containing contraception.
> - Progesterone contraception is not contraindicated if there is a thrombosis risk.
> - Long-acting reversible contraceptives (LARC), such as the levonorgestrel intrauterine system or progestogen implant, are effective and popular.

CASE 97: UNPROTECTED INTERCOURSE

History

A 24-year-old woman presents reporting a split condom during intercourse 22 h ago. She is now worried about pregnancy.

Her last menstrual period started 10 days ago and she has a regular 28-day menstrual cycle. She has never been pregnant in the past. She has been with this partner for the last 6 weeks. She is generally healthy with no relevant previous medical history although is overweight with a BMI of 31 kg/m².

Examination

Abdominal examination is unremarkable and internal examination is not indicated.

 INVESTIGATIONS

Urinary pregnancy test: Negative

? **QUESTIONS**

- What can you advise or offer this woman in regard to her concern about avoiding pregnancy?
- What other considerations are there in your clinical care apart from those relating to possible unplanned pregnancy and how would you deal with these?

ANSWER 97

This woman needs to be advised regarding emergency contraceptive options but first you must ascertain whether there is a risk that she may already be pregnant (from any other recent episodes of unprotected intercourse).

Although the pregnancy test is negative, if she had become pregnant in the last 2 weeks then she could be at the implantation stage, without the urinary human chorionic gonadotrophin (hCG) level being high enough to result in a positive urinary pregnancy test. This is known as a luteal phase pregnancy.

In this particular case, however, a luteal phase pregnancy is very unlikely as the last period was only 10 days ago and therefore ovulation would not yet be expected.

The options for the woman for emergency contraception with risks and benefits are listed below.

Emergency Contraceptive Pill

This is taken as a single tablet as soon as possible after unprotected intercourse. The single 1.5 mg levonorgestrel preparation is licensed for use for up to 72 h after intercourse and the single 30 mg ulipristal acetate preparation is licensed for 120 h after intercourse.

The emergency pill prevents pregnancy in 97–99 per cent of women and this is thought to be by inhibiting ovulation. However, it does not prevent pregnancies from subsequent unprotected sex in the same cycle.

There are no absolute medical contraindications for the emergency contraceptive pill, but drug interactions are possible so it should generally not be taken by women taking enzyme-inducing drugs and ulipristal acetate should not be used in women taking drugs that increase the gastric pH, such as antacids.

A few women vomit within 2 h after the emergency contraceptive pill, in which case they should be offered a further dose or the copper-bearing intrauterine device.

Emergency Intrauterine Contraceptive Device (IUCD)

The standard copper-bearing intrauterine device ('coil') can be inserted up to 5 days after sexual intercourse or up to 5 days after the earliest expected date of ovulation, whichever is the later. It should be left until at least the onset of the next period.

The IUCD is the most effective emergency contraceptive, preventing over 99 per cent of pregnancies, but may be associated with pain on or after insertion as well as risk of infection. Prophylactic antibiotics should therefore be considered at insertion. The advantage of this method of emergency contraception is that it provides ongoing contraception for as long as necessary until the device needs changing (usually 5 years).

> **!** **FACTORS INFLUENCING THE CHOICE OF EMERGENCY CONTRACEPTION**
>
> - Efficacy of method
> - Last menstrual period and cycle length
> - Number and timing of episodes of unprotected intercourse
> - Previous emergency contraceptive use within cycle (ulipristal acetate can only be used once per cycle)
> - Need for additional precautions/ongoing contraception
> - Drug interactions
> - Individual choice

Whichever emergency contraceptive method is used, the woman should be advised to take a pregnancy test in 3 weeks if a normal period has not occurred.

Non-Contraceptive Concerns

A woman who has had unprotected intercourse is at risk of sexually transmitted infection. Investigation with genital swabs at the time of first presentation should be considered for pre-existing infection. She should however be advised to be tested for chlamydia and gonorrhoea infection again after 3 weeks or longer for blood-borne infections such as hepatitis B and HIV.

Ongoing contraceptive needs should also always be discussed with any woman requesting emergency contraception.

 KEY POINTS

- Remember that a pregnancy conceived at the time of ovulation (day 14) will only register as a positive pregnancy test from around day 25.
- The copper intrauterine contraceptive device (inserted within 5 days of intercourse) is more effective at preventing pregnancy than the emergency contraceptive progestogen pill.

CASE 98: VAGINAL DISCHARGE

History

A 19-year-old woman presents with a vaginal discharge. She is currently 9 weeks pregnant in her first pregnancy. The discharge started about 3 weeks ago and is non-itchy and creamy in colour. It is not profuse but she feels it has a strong odour and is embarrassed about it. There is no bleeding or abdominal pain. She has had two or three previous similar episodes before the pregnancy and these resolved spontaneously.

She has been with her partner for 3 years and neither of them have had any other sexual partners. They always used condoms until 3 months ago. She has never had a cervical smear test.

Examination

The external genitalia appear normal. On speculum examination a small amount of smooth grey discharge is seen coating the vagina walls. There is a small cervical ectropion that is not bleeding.

? | **QUESTIONS**

- What is the likely diagnosis and the differential diagnosis?
- How would you further investigate and manage this patient?
- If your diagnosis is confirmed, what are the implications for the pregnancy?

DOI: 10.1201/9781003386933-104

ANSWER 98

The history suggests that the woman is not at risk of a sexually transmitted infection as a cause for her discharge (although this can never be ruled out entirely as the reported sexual history can be inaccurate). She has an ectropion, which can cause a clear discharge. A nonoffensive, non-itchy discharge is normal in pregnancy.

The salient feature in this case is that the discharge has an offensive odour. Offensive odour is usually due to either trichomonas or bacterial vaginosis (BV). Trichomonas causes a profuse, sometimes frothy discharge with cervicitis, whereas BV causes a smooth, mild discharge, if any discharge at all.

Differential Diagnosis of Vaginal Discharge

- *Infective*:
  - Sexually transmitted: Trichomonas, chlamydia, gonorrhoea
  - Non-sexually transmitted: Candida, bacterial vaginosis
- *Physiological*:
  - Pregnancy
  - Ovulation
- Cervical ectropion

Further Investigation

The woman should have swabs taken for sexually transmitted infection as well as BV and candida. A diagnosis of BV can be made by the finding of a typical thin grey discharge with a fishy odour and a vaginal pH of >4.5. More formal criteria for diagnosis are the Amsel (discharge, clue cells on microscopy, high pH and fishy odour with potassium hydroxide) or Hay/Ison (relative lactobacilli to anaerobe proportions on Gram-stained vaginal smear) criteria. Microbiological culture is not helpful as many of the anaerobes associated with BV are also found as commensals.

Management

Spontaneous onset and remission are typical with BV, and 50 per cent of women are asymptomatic. General advice should be given for avoiding BV including avoidance of vaginal douching, shower gel and antiseptic agents or shampoo in the bath, as these interfere with the normal flora (lactobacilli) and allow an increase in BV organisms. Specific treatment is with vaginal clindamycin cream or oral metronidazole for 5–7 days.

BV and Pregnancy

Late miscarriage, preterm birth, preterm premature rupture of membranes, and postpartum endometritis have all been associated with BV, and so any pregnant woman with BV should be treated with clindamycin or metronidazole. In contrast, non-pregnant women only require treatment if symptomatic.

 KEY POINTS

- BV is a common cause of discharge and is the most likely diagnosis in a woman complaining of an offensive or fishy odour, but a full sexually transmitted infection screen is usually indicated to rule out other co-existing infection.
- Treatment with clindamycin or metronidazole is indicated in all affected pregnant women, but in non-pregnant women it is only indicated for those with symptoms.

CASE 99: TEENAGE CONTRACEPTION

History

A 14-year-old girl attends a family planning clinic wanting to start 'the pill'. She has been with her boyfriend for 8 months. They both agreed that they wanted to start a sexual relationship and have already had intercourse on two occasions where they did not use contraception. She had never been sexually active before. Her periods started 3 years ago and were initially irregular but she now reports a regular 27-day cycle. She has never had any gynaecological or other medical problems.

She reports that she is happy at school and she is one of three children, with a brother of 21 and sister of 19 years. She lives with her parents in a house locally. She has attended the clinic with a female school friend.

Examination

There are no examination or investigations findings.

? | **QUESTIONS**

- What issues are important in determining how this situation should be managed?
- How would you further investigate, advise and manage the situation in this scenario?

DOI: 10.1201/9781003386933-105

ANSWER 99

Prescribing of contraception to girls under the legal age of consent (16 years) is guided by the Fraser rules, which arose from the case of Gillick seeking to stop a doctor from providing contraceptive advice to her daughter without consulting the parents.

The law allows contraception to be provided as long as the following criteria are met:

- The girl should be encouraged to discuss her sexual activity with a parent or another responsible adult.
- She should consent to intercourse.
- She should understand the implications of having sexual intercourse and the contraceptive method chosen.
- It is anticipated that she will have sex whether or not contraception is provided and is therefore at potentially higher physical and psychological harm from an inadvertent pregnancy.

In this case it is clear that the girl will continue to have sex with or without contraception as she has already done so, and therefore it is in her best interests to prevent pregnancy. She should be encouraged to discuss the issue with a parent, or failing this perhaps her older sister or brother.

The age of her boyfriend should be explored – if he is of a similar age then consent is probably valid. However if there is a significant age discrepancy, e.g. he was over 20 years, then issues of child protection should be considered and the case should be discussed in the first instance with a member of the safeguarding team.

Investigation and Advice

A urinary pregnancy test should be performed prior to giving any hormonal contraception, as she has already had unprotected intercourse and could already be pregnant.

She should be advised about the different methods of contraception, particularly how to use them and the importance of compliance. The availability of emergency contraception should be explained.

She is at risk of sexually transmitted infections, and barrier contraception should be advised even if she is using a contraceptive pill or other method as her main pregnancy-prevention strategy.

Whichever option is chosen, the girl should be supported such that she is happy to come back for further review and to check correct usage of the preferred method. Explanation of confidentiality rules will also aid her confidence in your advice.

 KEY POINTS

- Contraception may be provided to girls under the age of 16 years without parental consent subject to the guidance in the Fraser rules.
- Sexually transmitted infections and education about emergency contraception are an integral part of such consultations.

CASE 100: INTERMENSTRUAL BLEEDING

History

A 21-year-old student presents with vaginal bleeding between her periods. It first occurred 2 months ago and she has had several recurrences. It is usually light and generally lasts from 1 to 3 days.

She has been using the combined oral contraceptive pill (COCP) for 18 months and has regular withdrawal bleeds, which occur every 28 days and last for 3 days. The withdrawal bleeds are not heavy or painful. She has not noticed any other vaginal discharge. She has not had any bowel or urinary symptoms.

She first had sexual intercourse at the age of 17 years and has been with her current boyfriend for 4 months. There is no pain on intercourse and no postcoital bleeding.

She was seen once before in the gynaecology clinic for pelvic pain and was noted to have a simple ovarian cyst, which subsequently resolved spontaneously. There is no other significant medical history of note. The general practitioner had arranged an ultrasound assessment prior to referral.

Examination

She is slim and looks well. The abdomen is not distended and is non-tender. The external genitalia are normal and on speculum examination a slight blood-stained discharge is noted coming from the cervical os. There is a cervical ectropion which is not bleeding on contact with the speculum.

Bimanual examination reveals an anteverted normal size mobile uterus. There is no cervical motion tenderness or adnexal tenderness.

 INVESTIGATIONS

Transvaginal ultrasound examination: The uterus is normal size and anteverted. The endometrium measures 7 mm in anteroposterior diameter and is regular along its entire length with no evidence of an endometrial polyp.
Both ovaries appear of normal size and morphology.
There is no free peritoneal fluid.
Urinary pregnancy test: Negative

? **QUESTIONS**

- What further questions would you like to ascertain answers to in the history?
- What is the differential diagnosis?
- How would you further investigate and manage this woman?

DOI: 10.1201/9781003386933-106

ANSWER 100

The symptom of bleeding between the pill-free intervals in a woman taking the combined oral contraceptive pill is known as breakthrough bleeding. It can have many causes and a good history should include, in addition to the history already given:

- Has she been missing any pills?
- Has she taken any other medication which might interfere with the COCP (e.g. antibiotics or enzyme inducers)?
- Has she had any intercurrent illnesses causing diarrhoea or vomiting?
- Has she ever had any sexually transmitted infections, or been investigated for this?
- How many sexual partners has she had in the last 3 months?
- Has she recently changed the COCP that she uses?

> ! **DIFFERENTIAL DIAGNOSIS IN A WOMAN WITH BREAKTHROUGH BLEEDING**
>
> - *COCP-related causes:*
>   - Poor compliance
>   - Intercurrent infection causing poor pill absorption
>   - Drug interactions, reducing the COCP efficacy
>   - Inadequate oestrogen component for that woman
>   - Pregnancy
> - *Unrelated causes:*
>   - Cervical ectropion
>   - Cervical carcinoma
>   - Sexually transmitted infection – chlamydia, gonorrhoea, trichomonas
>   - Candida vaginitis
>   - Cervical or endometrial polyp
>   - Bleeding disorder (rare)

A cervical ectropion is very common in young women, especially when using the COCP. It can be a cause of unscheduled (usually postcoital) bleeding but in this case there was no bleeding on contact with the speculum and so it should be considered an incidental finding.

The woman should have the following swabs taken:

- *Endocervical* – for chlamydia
- *High vaginal* – for trichomonas or candida
- *Endocervical* – for gonorrhoea

(Bacterial vaginosis is another vaginal infection but does not cause bleeding.)

Chlamydia is a common sexually transmitted infection, especially in women aged 18–24 years. It is often asymptomatic or may present with minimal symptoms as in this case. It should be tested for with an endocervical swab, though urine testing and low vaginal swab testing are also possible. If confirmed, the woman should be treated with doxycycline, azithromycin or erythromycin (dependent on local guidelines, allergies and chance of possible pregnancy) and advised that her partner(s) should also be tested and treated at a sexual health clinic before they resume intercourse.

Chlamydia may cause ascending pelvic infection and subsequent tubal factor infertility, as well as increasing the chance of ectopic pregnancy in future, so compliance needs to be encouraged.

If the swabs are negative and no other cause can be identified for the breakthrough bleeding, then the woman should be changed to an alternative combined contraceptive pill. There is no one formulation to suit all women, and a trial and error approach is needed. Possibilities include a preparation with a different second or third generation progestogen (avoiding norethisterone which can be associated with more breakthrough bleeding) or a pill containing a higher dose of oestrogen (such as 30 mg rather than 20 mg). Extended or continuous use of the pill may also be tried.

 KEY POINTS

- Breakthrough bleeding with the combined oral contraceptive pill can have many causes.
- Chlamydia infection is often asymptomatic or presents with vague symptoms such as irregular bleeding.
- Compliance with medication, contact tracing and avoidance of sexual intercourse until completion of treatment by both partners is essential in the management of chlamydia infection.

INDEX